PATHOLOGY PRACTICAL BOOK

for Dental Students

The photographs on the cover of the textbook depict images of diseases as follows:

Aspergillosis lung,
Gomori's methenamine silver (GMS) stain

Megaloblastic anaemia,
Bone marrow aspirate

Fibroadenoma breast, FNA
MGG stain

Metastatic carcinoma lymph node,
H & E stain

PATHOLOGY PRACTICAL BOOK
for Dental Students

Harsh Mohan MD, FAMS, FICPath, FUICC
Professor and Head
Department of Pathology
Government Medical College
Sector-32 A, Chandigarh-160 031
INDIA
E mail: drharshmohan@gmail.com

Sugandha Mohan BDS
E mail: sugandha1987@gmail.com

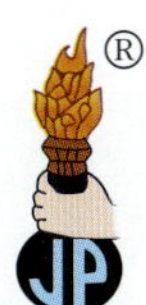

JAYPEE BROTHERS MEDICAL PUBLISHERS (P) LTD
New Delhi • Panama City • London

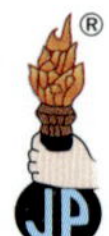

Jaypee Brothers Medical Publishers (P) Ltd.

Headquarter

Jaypee Brothers Medical Publishers (P) Ltd
4838/24, Ansari Road, Daryaganj
New Delhi 110 002, India
Phone: +91-11-43574357
Fax: +91-11-43574314
Email: jaypee@jaypeebrothers.com

Overseas Offices

J.P. Medical Ltd.,
83 Victoria Street London
SW1H 0HW (UK)
Phone: +44-2031708910
Fax: +02-03-0086180
Email: info@jpmedpub.com

Jaypee-Highlights Medical Publishers Inc.
City of Knowledge, Bld. 237, Clayton
Panama City, Panama
Phone: 507-317-0160
Fax: +50-73-010499
Email: cservice@jphmedical.com

Website: www.jaypeebrothers.com
Website: www.jaypeedigital.com

Inquiries for bulk sales may be solicited at: jaypee@jaypeebrothers.com

Publisher: Jitendar P Vij
Publishing Director: Tarun Duneja
Assistant Editors: Praveen Mohan, Tanya Mohan
Cover Design: Seema Dogra, Sumit Kumar

Pathology Practical Book for Dental Students

First Edition: **2012**

ISBN 978-93-5025-495-0

Printed at Replika Press Pvt. Ltd.

Preface

न हि ज्ञानेन सदृभाम् पवित्रम् इह विद्यते ।
तत् स्वयम् योगसंसिद्धः कालेन आत्मनि विन्दति ।।

There is nothing in this world
Equal in purity to knowledge,
And the one who has perfected by practice
Enjoys this knowledge in due course of time.

(The Bhagvatgita: Ch IV, Verse 38)

Students of dentistry in India (and in many other countries) learn pathology in two phases—General Pathology in second year and Oral Pathology in their third year of the course. As an experienced teacher (HM) and as a BDS student until recently (SM), it has been our common observation that BDS students who are studying in shared campuses for BDS and MBBS, get much less attention from their teachers of medical college in general medical subjects than the attention and care they get from their teachers of core dental subjects from their dentistry teachers for various reasons which we are not delving into. Similarly, until a few years back, there were no separate books in general medical subjects taught to dental students. Thus, while there has been a main course book *Essential Pathology for Dental Students* by the first author for about 15 years, there has not been any separate practical book in pathology for BDS students so far anywhere. This has resulted in lack of uniformity in teaching and training for the reason that it is left to the discretion of teacher and examiner to decide what to teach and evaluate and what to leave out for dental students.

An attempt has been made to bridge this lacuna by bringing out separately the present book, *Pathology Practical Book for Dental Students,* structured as per requirements prescribed by the Dental Council of India (DCI) in the revised syllabus of Pathology for second year BDS students.

Some *highlights* of this book are as under:

Updated and well-organised contents: The book is organised systematically into 4 Sections, each section having certain number of practical exercises (in all 25) patterned on the format of practical class of students. These are: Techniques in Pathology (Exercise 1-4), Clinical Pathology and Basic Cytopathology (Exercise 5-7), Haematology (Exercise 8-13) and Histopathology (Exercise 14-25).

Hone your diagnostic skills: The book is structured in a way that it aims to hone the practical and diagnostic skills of the learner in pathology in a user-friendly manner. All exercises have listed key features point-wise for easy understanding and reproducibility, leaving out theoretical details for learning from the main course book so as not to lose focus on key diagnostic and practical points.

Brevity with beauty: Brief and point-wise text in each exercise is richly supported by labelled line-drawings with corresponding specimen photograph and microscopic image for conceptual learning. Thus, the book may become a must-take to practical class by the students to learn the subject effectively and to revise the entire matter quickly for their examination and viva.

Wish to learn more? For those students desiring to learn more, the book has many additional exercises over and above those given in the revised syllabus by the DCI in the opening pages of the book.

Although the book is primarily prepared as per DCI recommendations given in the revised syllabus in Pathology for second year students of BDS, it is also expected to be useful for practising clinicians and other students of medicine such as those pursuing course in physiotherapy, pharmacy, nursing, laboratory technology and alternate systems of medicine.

In preparing this book, we have been helped and supported by various friends and colleagues and our family, which is gratefully acknowledged. A word of special thanks to Ms Agam Verma, MSc (MLT), Senior Laboratory Technician, for liberal and skilful technical assistance and her valuable suggestions in chapters on laboratory technology.

We thank profusely the entire staff of M/s Jaypee Brothers Medical Publishers (P) Ltd. for their ever smiling support and cooperation in completion of this book in a relatively short time.

Finally, although sincere effort has been made to be as accurate as possible, element of human error is still likely; we shall humbly request users to continue giving their valuable suggestions and feedback directed at further improvements of its contents.

Government Medical College
Sector-32 A, Chandigarh-160030
INDIA

Harsh Mohan MD, FAMS, FICPath, FUICC
Professor and Head
Department of Pathology
E mail: drharshmohan@gmail.com

Sugandha Mohan BDS
E mail: sugandha1987@gmail.com

Contents

Revised Syllabus in Pathology for BDS Students as per Recommendations of the Dental Council of India

COURSE CONTENTS IN PRACTICAL

Urine—Abnormal Constituents: Sugar, albumin, ketone bodies.

Urine—Abnormal Constituents: Blood, bile salts, bile pigments.

Haemoglobin (Hb) Estimation

Total WBC Count

Differential WBC Count

Packed Cell Volume (PCV), Erythrocyte Sedimentation Rate (ESR)

Bleeding Time and Clotting Time

Histopathology: Tissue processing, staining.

Histopathology Slides:

- Acute appendicitis, granulation tissue, fatty liver.
- CVC lung, CVC liver, amyloidosis kidney.
- Tuberculosis, actinomycosis, rhinosporidiosis.
- Papilloma, basal cell carcinoma, squamous cell carcinoma.
- Osteosarcoma, osteoclastoma, fibrosarcoma.
- Malignant melanoma, ameloblastoma, adenoma.
- Mixed parotid tumour, metastatic carcinoma in lymph node.

Section One

TECHNIQUES IN PATHOLOGY

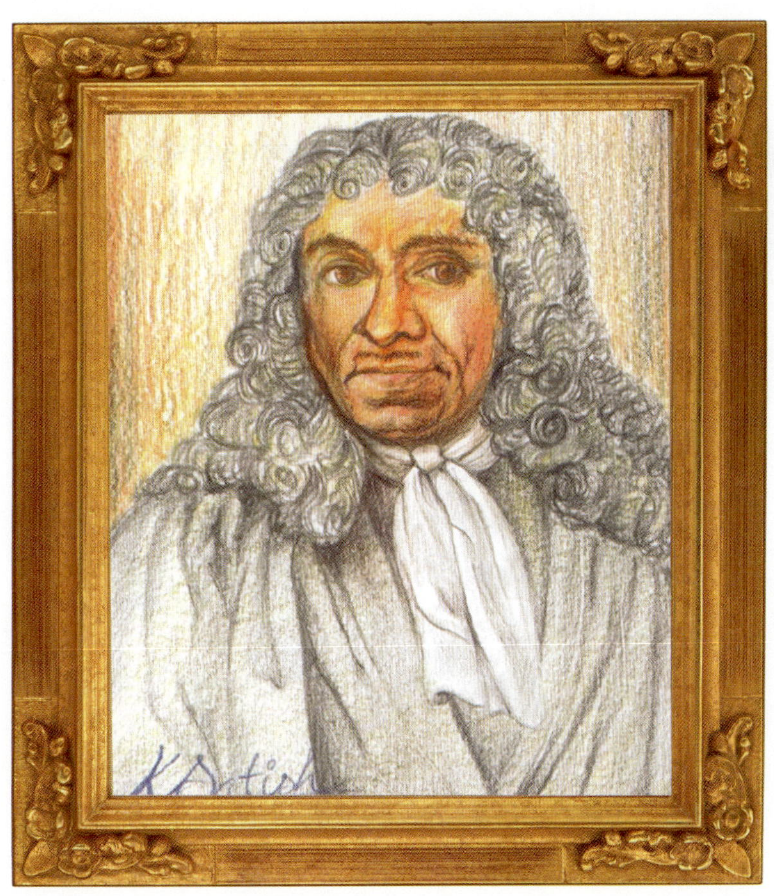

ANTHONY VAN LEEUWENHOEK (1632–1723)

Born in Holland, draper by profession, during his spare time invented the first ever microscope by grinding the lenses himself and made 400 microscopes. He also first introduced histological staining in 1714 by using saffron to examine muscle fibre.

Section Contents

Exercise

1

Microscopy of Various Types

Objectives

- Describe the working of various parts of a light microscope. How do we maintain and operate a light microscope?
- Enumerate various other types of microscopy, mentioning their broad principles.

Microscope is the most commonly used piece of apparatus in the laboratory. It produces magnified images of minute objects.

Common light microscope is described first, followed by other special types of microscopy techniques.

LIGHT MICROSCOPE

A light microscope can be a simple or a compound microscope.

Simple microscope This is a simple hand magnifying lens. The magnification power of hand lens is from 2x to 200x.

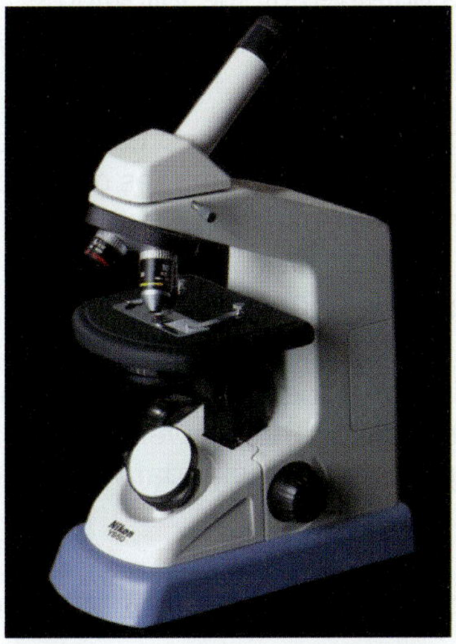

FIGURE 1.1: Monocular light microscope, Model YS 50 (Photograph courtesy of Nikon, Japan through Towa Optics India Pvt. Ltd., Delhi).

Compound microscope This has a battery of lenses which are fitted in a complex instrument. One type of lens remains near the object *(objective lens)* and another type of lens near the observer's eye *(eyepiece lens).* The eyepiece and objective lenses have different magnification. The compound microscope can be *monocular* having single eyepiece (Fig. 1.1) or, *binocular* which has two eyepieces (Fig. 1.2). The usual type of microscope used in clinical laboratories is called compound microscope.

A compound microscope has the following parts:

- Stand
- Body

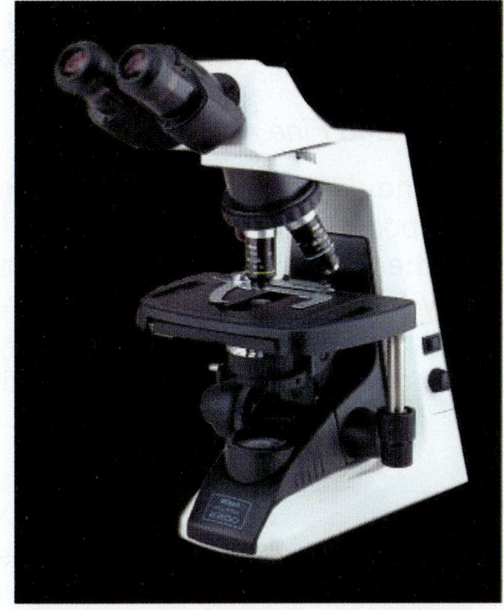

FIGURE 1.2: Binocular light microscope, Model E 200 (Photograph courtesy of Nikon, Japan through Towa Optics India Pvt. Ltd., Delhi).

- Optical system
- Light/illumination system

Stand

This is horse-shoe shaped in monocular microscope. It gives stability to the microscope. Binocular microscopes have a variety of ergonomic shapes of stand.

Body

It consists of a limb which arises from the joint with which microscope can be moved in comfortable position. The stand and the limb carry the following:

i. Body tubes
ii. Stage
iii. Knobs for coarse and fine adjustment

Body Tubes

There are two tubes: *external tube* which carries at its lower end a revolving nosepiece having objective lenses of different magnification while *internal tube* is draw tube which carries at its upper end eyepieces.

Stage

This is a metallic platform which accommodates glass slide having mounted object over it to be seen. Stage is attached to the limb just below the level of objectives. It has an aperture in its centre which permits the light to reach the object. Slide on the stage can be moved horizontally or vertically by two knobs attached to slide holder. Just below the stage is *substage* which consists of condenser through which light is focused on the object. The substage can be moved up and down. The substage has an iris diaphragm, closing and opening of which controls the amount of light reaching the object.

Knobs for Coarse and Fine Adjustment

For coarse and fine adjustments, knobs are provided on either side of the body. Coarse adjustment has two bigger knobs, one on the either side, the movement of which moves the body tubes with its lenses. Fine adjustment has two smaller knobs on either side of the body. The fine focus is graduated and by each division objective moves by 0.002 mm.

Optical System

Optical system is comprised by different lenses which are fitted into a microscope. It consists of eyepiece, objectives and condensers.

Eyepiece

In monocular microscope, there is one eyepiece while binocular microscope has two. Eyepiece has two plano-convex lenses. Their magnification can be 5x, 10x, or 15x.

Objectives

These are made of a battery of lenses with prisms incorporated in them. Their magnification power is 4x, 10x, 40x and 100x.

Condenser

This is made up of two simple lenses and it condenses light on to the object.

Light/Illumination System

For daylight illumination, a mirror is fitted which is plane on one side and concave on the other side (Fig. 1.1). Plane mirror is used in sunlight while concave in artificial light. Currently, most of the microscopes have in-built electrical illumination varying from 20 to 100 watts (Fig. 1.2).

Magnification and Resolving Power of Light Microscope

Magnification power of the microscope is the degree of image enlargement. It depends upon the following:

i. Length of optical tube
ii. Magnifying power of objective
iii. Magnifying power of eyepiece

With a fixed tube length of 160 mm in majority of standard microscopes, the magnification power of the microscope is obtained by the following:

Magnifying power of objective × Magnifying power of eyepiece.

Resolving power represents the capacity of the optical system to produce separate images of objects very close to each other and is obtained as under:

$$\text{Resolving power (R)} = \frac{0.61\,\lambda}{\text{NA}}$$

Where λ is wavelength of incidental light; and
NA is numerical aperture of lens.

Resolving power of a standard light microscope is around 200 nm.

How to Use and Maintain a Light Microscope

1. Keep the microscope in comfortable position.

2. Obtain appropriate illumination by adjusting the mirror or intensity of light.
3. When examining colourless objects, condenser should be at the lowest position and iris diaphragm closed or partially closed.
4. When using oil immersion, 100x objective should dip in oil.
5. After using oil immersion clean the lens of the objective with tissue paper or soft cloth.

OTHER TYPES OF MICROSCOPY

Dark Ground Illumination (DGI)

This method is used for examination of unstained living micro-organisms e.g. *Treponema pallidum.*

Principle

The micro-organisms are illuminated by an oblique ray of light which does not pass through the micro-organism. The condenser is blackened in the centre and light passes through its periphery illuminating the living micro-organism on a glass slide.

Polarising Microscope

This method is used for demonstration of birefringence e.g. amyloid, foreign body, hair etc.

Principle

The light is made plane polarised. Two discs made up of prism are placed in the path of light, one below the object known as *polariser* and another placed in the body tube which is known as *analyser.* Polariser sieves out ordinary light rays vibrating in all directions allowing light waves of one orientation to pass through. The lower disc (polariser) is rotated to make the light plane polarised. During rotation, when analyser comes perpendicular to polariser, all light rays are cancelled or extinguished. Birefringent objects rotate the light rays and therefore appear bright in a dark background.

Fluorescent Microscope

This method is used for demonstration of naturally-occurring fluorescent material and other non-fluorescent substances or micro-organisms after staining than with some fluorescent dyes e.g. *Mycobacterium tuberculosis*, amyloid, lipids, elastic fibres etc. UV light is used for illumination.

Principle

Fluorescent microscopy depends upon illumination of a substance with a specific higher wavelength (UV region i.e. invisible region) which then emits light at a lower wavelength (visible region).

Electron Microscope (EM)

EM is used to study ultrastructural details of the tissues and cells. For electron microscopy, tissue is fixed in 4% glutaraldehyde at 4°C for 4 hours. Ultrathin microsections with thickness of 100 nm are cut with diamond knives.

Principle

By using an electron beam of light, the resolving power of the microscope is increased to 50,000 to 100,000 times and very small structures can be visualised. In contrast to light microscopy, resolution of electron microscopy is 0.2 nm or less.

There are two types of electron microscopy:

1. Transmission electron microscopy (TEM)
2. Scanning electron microscopy (SEM)

Transmission Electron Microscopy (TEM)

TEM helps visualise cell's cytoplasm and organelles. For this purpose, ultrathin sections are required. TEM interprets atomic rather than molecular properties of the tissue and gives two dimensional image of the tissue.

Scanning Electron Microscopy (SEM)

SEM helps in the study of cell surface. In this three-dimensional image is produced. The image is produced on cathode ray oscillograph which can also be amplified. SEM can also be used for fluorescent antibody techniques.

Exercise

2

Histopathology Techniques and Routine Staining

Objectives

- Discuss fixation of tissues and principles of common fixatives used in a tissue laboratory.
- Describe basic technique of routine histopathology processing of tissues in the laboratory and various equipments used for it.
- Discuss the technique of routine H and E staining of tissues.

Histology is the science of examination of normal tissues at microscopic level. Histopathology is examination of tissues for presence or absence of changes in their structure due to disease processes. Both are done by examining thin sections of tissues which are coloured differently by different dyes and stains. Total or selected representative part of tissue not more than 4 mm thick is placed in steel or plastic capsules or cassettes and is subjected to the following sequential steps (tissue processing):

- Fixation
- Dehydration, Clearing, Impregnation } *Processing*
- Embedding and blocking
- Section cutting (Microtomy)
- Routine staining (H & E)

FIXATION

Any tissue removed from the body starts decomposing immediately because of loss of blood supply and oxygen, accumulation of products of metabolism, action of autolytic enzymes and putrefaction by bacteria. This process of decomposition is prevented by fixation. Fixation is the method of preserving cells and tissues in life-like conditions as far as possible. During fixation, tissues are fixed in complete physical and partly chemical state. Most fixatives act by denaturation or precipitation of cell proteins or by making soluble components of cell insoluble. Fixative produces the following *effects:*

i. Prevents putrefaction and autolysis.
ii. Hardens the tissue which helps in section cutting.
iii. Makes cell insensitive to hypertonic or hypotonic solutions.
iv. Acts as a mordant.
v. Induces optical contrast for good morphologic examination.

An ideal fixative has the following properties:

i. It should be cheap and easily available.
ii. It should be stable and safe to handle.
iii. It should be rapid in action.
iv. It should cause minimal loss of tissue.
v. It should not bind to the reactive groups in tissue which are meant for dyes.
vi. It should give even penetration.
vii. It should retain normal colour of the tissue.

Types of Fixatives

Fixatives may be simple or compound:

- *Simple fixative* consists of one substance (e.g. formalin).
- *Compound fixative* has two or more substances (e.g. Bouin's, Zenker's).

Fixatives can also be divided into following 3 groups:

- *Microanatomical fixatives* which preserve the anatomy of the tissue.
- *Cytological fixatives* which may be cytoplasmic or nuclear and preserve respective intracellular constituents.
- *Histochemical fixatives* employed for demonstration of histochemical constituents and enzymes.

Commonly used fixatives are as under:

1. Formalin
2. Glutaraldehyde
3. Picric acid (e.g. Bouin's fluid)
4. Alcohol (e.g. Carnoy's fixative)
5. Osmium tetraoxide

1. Formalin

This is the most commonly used fixative in routine practice. Formalin is commercially available as saturated solution of formaldehyde gas in water, 40% by weight/volume (w/v). For all practical purposes, this 40% solution is considered as 100% formalin. For routine fixation, 10% formalin is used which is prepared by dissolving 10 ml of commercially available formalin in 90 ml of water. Duration of fixation depends upon size and thickness of tissue, type of tissue and its density. It takes 6-8 hours for fixation of a thin piece of tissue 4 mm thick at room temperature. The amount of fixative should be 15 to 20 times the volume of the specimen. Formalin acts by polymerisation of cellular proteins by forming methylene bridges between protein molecules.

Merits of formalin

1. Rapidly penetrates the tissues.
2. Normal colour of tissue is retained.
3. It is cheap and easily available.
4. It is the best fixative for neurological tissue.

Demerits of formalin

1. Causes excessive hardening of tissues.
2. Causes irritation of skin, mucous membranes and conjunctiva.
3. Leads to formation of formalin pigment in tissues having excessive blood at an acidic pH which can be removed by treatment of section with alcoholic picric acid.

2. Glutaraldehyde

This is used as a fixative in electron microscopy. Glutaraldehyde is used as 4% solution at 4°C for 4 hours for fixation of tissues.

Disadvantages of glutaraldehyde

1. It is expensive.
2. It penetrates the tissues slowly.

3. Bouin's Fluid (Picric acid)

This is used as fixative for renal and testicular needle biopsies. Bouin's fluid stains the tissues yellow. It is also a good fixative for demonstration of glycogen. It is prepared as under:

Saturated picric acid	-	375 ml
40% formaldehyde	-	125 ml
Glacial acetic acid	-	25 ml

Disadvantages

1. Makes the tissue harder and brittle.
2. Causes lysis of RBCs.

4. Carnoy's Fixative (Alcohol)

Alcohol is mainly used for fixation of cytologic smears and endometrial curettings. It acts by denaturation of cell proteins. Both methyl and ethyl alcohol can be used. Methyl alcohol is used as 100% solution for 20-30 minutes. Ethyl alcohol is used either as 95% solution or as Carnoy's fixative for tissues which contains the following:

Ethyl alcohol (absolute)	-	300 ml
Chloroform	-	150 ml
Glacial acetic acid	-	50 ml

Carnoy's is a good fixative for glycogen and dissolves fat.

5. Osmium Tetraoxide

This is used as a fixative for CNS tissues and for electron microscopy. Osmium tetraoxide is best fixative for lipids. It is used as a 2% solution. It imparts black colour to tissues.

DEHYDRATION

This is a process in which water from the tissues and cells is removed so that this space so created is subsequently taken up by wax. Dehydration is carried out by passing the tissues through a series of ascending grades of alcohol: 70%, 80%, 95% and absolute alcohol. If ethyl alcohol is not available, other alternatives such as methyl alcohol, isopropyl alcohol or acetone can be used.

CLEARING

This is the process in which alcohol from the tissues and cells is removed (dealcoholisation) and is replaced by a fluid in which wax is soluble. It also makes the tissue transparent. Xylene is the most commonly used clearing agent. Toluene, benzene (it is carcinogenic), chloroform (it is poisonous) and cedar wood oil (it is expensive and very viscous) can also be used as clearing agents.

IMPREGNATION

This is the process in which empty spaces in the tissues and cells after removal of clearing agent are taken up molten by paraffin wax. This hardens the tissue which helps in section cutting. Impregnation is done in molten paraffin wax which has the melting point ranging from 54-62°C.

TISSUE PROCESSORS

Nowadays, processes of dehydration, clearing and impregnation are carried out in a composite equipment which is known as *automated tissue processor.* It can be an open (hydraulic) system or a closed (vacuum) type.

Open (Hydraulic) Tissue Processor

It has 12 stations—10 stations are glass/steel jars and 2 stations have thermostatically controlled wax bath. These jars are used as follow:

- For *fixation* in formalin: 1 jar.
- For *dehydration* in ascending grades of alcohol: 6 jars, one each of 70%, 80%, 90% and 3 for 100%.
- For *clearing* in xylene: 3 jars.
- For *impregnation* in molten paraffin wax: 2 wax baths.

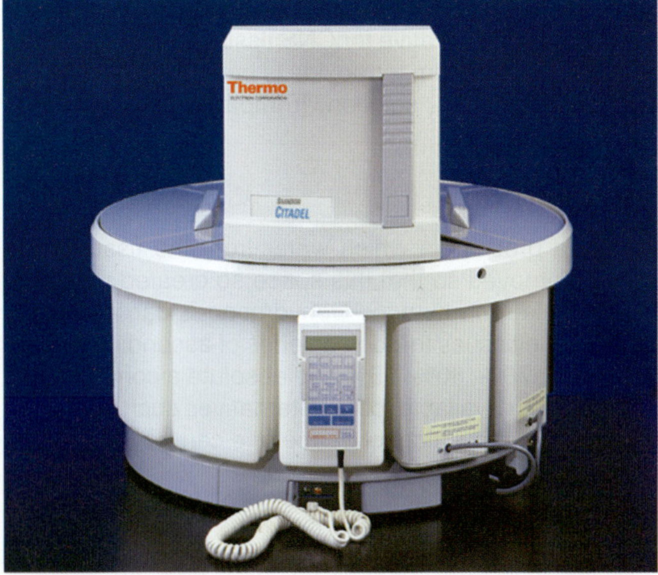

FIGURE 2.1: Automatic tissue processor (Photograph courtesy of Thermo Shandon, UK through Towa Optics India Pvt. Ltd., Delhi).

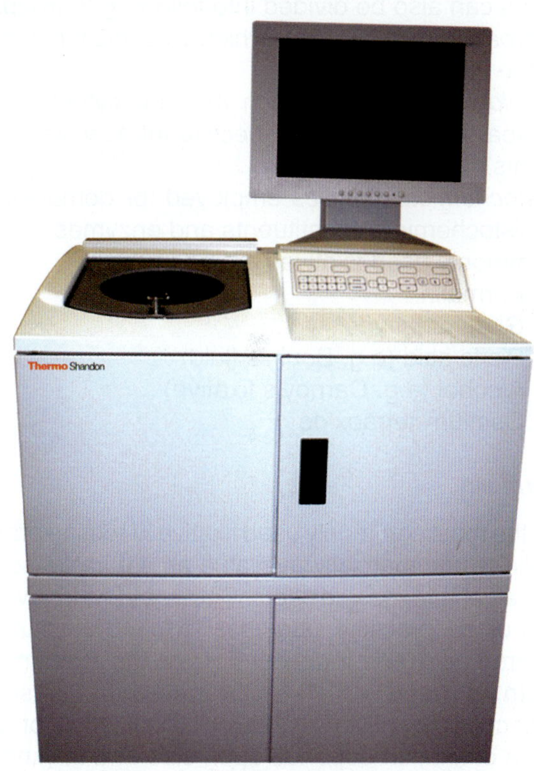

FIGURE 2.2: Vacuum tissue processor, Model Excelsior (Photograph courtesy of Thermo Shandon, UK through Towa Optics Pvt. Ltd., Delhi).

Tissue moves automatically by hydraulic mechanism from one jar to the next after fixed time schedule as set in the program (Fig. 2.1). Generally, 1.5 hours duration is given at each station and whole process takes about 18 hours (overnight). For rapid processing, modern systems have programs for short run in which entire tissue processing is completed in maximum of 2.5 hours; tissue stays at each stations for 10-20 minutes. Nowadays, modifications are available in which vacuum system can be incorporated in open (hydraulic) types.

Closed (Vacuum) Tissue Processor

In the closed type of tissue processor, tissue cassettes are placed in a single container while different processing fluids are moved in and out sequentially according to electronically programmed cycle (Fig. 2.2). The closed or vacuum processor has the advantage that there is no hazard of contamination of the laboratory by toxic fumes unlike in open system. In addition, heat and vacuum shorten the processing time. Thus, closed tissue processors can also be applied for short schedules or rapid processing of small biopsies.

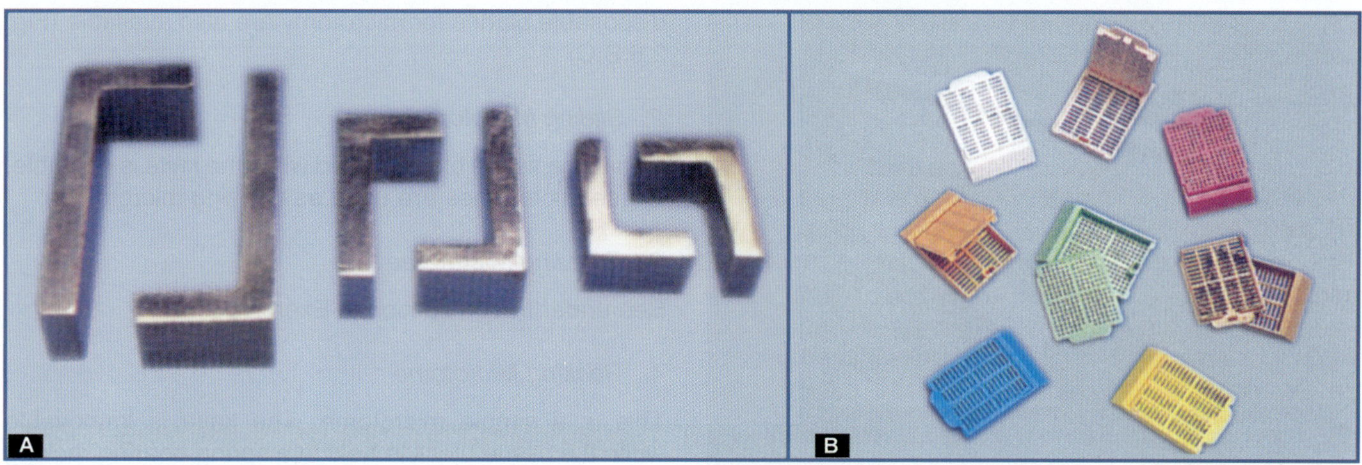

FIGURE 2.3: A, L (Leuckhart's) metal moulds. B, Plastic block moulds in different colours.

EMBEDDING AND BLOCKING

Embedding of tissue is done in molten wax. Wax blocks can be conventionally prepared using metallic L (Leuckhart's) moulds; nowadays plastic moulds of different colours for blocking are also available (Fig. 2.3). The moulds are placed over a smooth surfaced glass tile. Molten wax is poured into the cavity in the moulds. The processed tissue pieces are put into wax with number tag and examining surface facing downward. Wax is allowed to solidify. After solidification, if L-moulds are used they are removed, while plastic mould remains with the wax block. In either case, each block contains a tissue piece carrying an identification label.

Embedding and blocking can also be performed in a special equipment called *embedding centre*. It has a wax reservoir, heated area for steel moulds, wax dispenser, and separate hot and cold plates for embedding and blocking (Fig. 2.4).

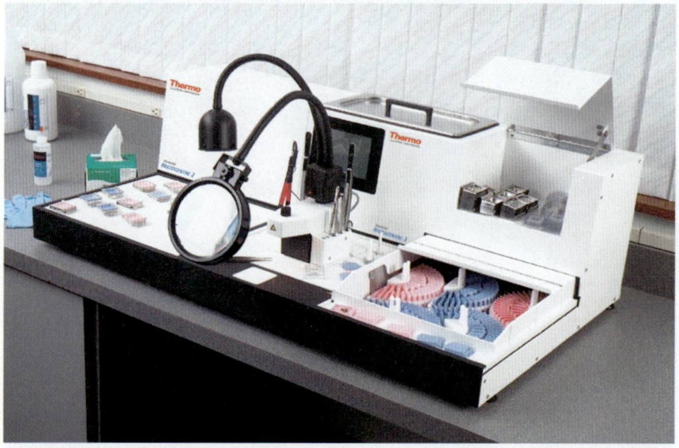

FIGURE 2.4: Tissue embedding centre, Model Histocentre (Photograph courtesy of Thermo Shandon, UK through Towa Optics (India) Pvt. Ltd., Delhi).

SECTION CUTTING (MICROTOMY)

Microtome is an equipment for cutting sections and the technique of section cutting is called microtomy. There are 5 types of microtomes:

1. Rotary
2. Sliding
3. Freezing
4. Rocking
5. Base-sledge

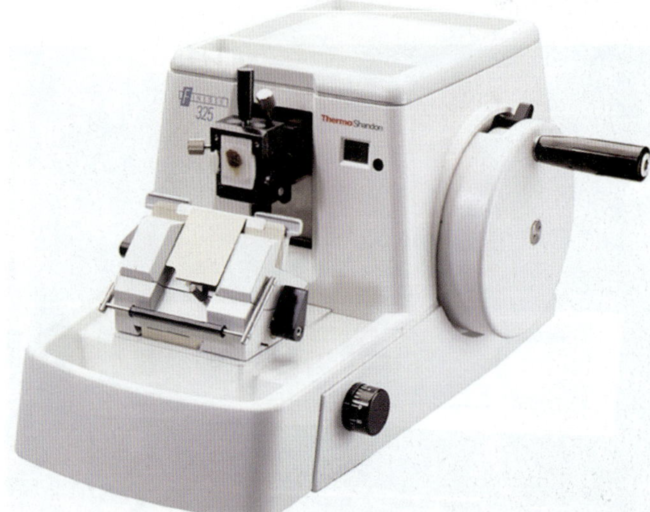

FIGURE 2.5: Rotary microtome, Model Finesse 325 (Photograph courtesy of Thermo Shandon, UK through Towa Optics India Pvt. Ltd., Delhi).

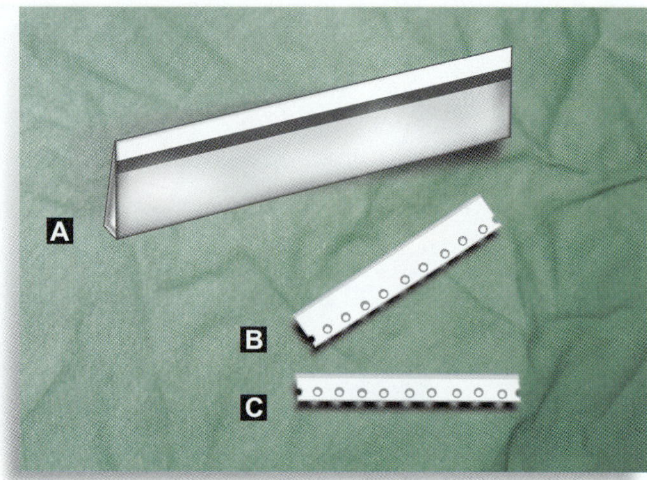

FIGURE 2.6: A, Plain wedge knife for rotary microtome. B,C, Disposable blades for microtomy—high profile type and low profile type respectively.

1. Rotary Microtome

This is the most commonly used microtome. In this, microtome knife is fixed while the tissue block is movable (Fig. 2.5). The knife used is of stainless steel and is wedge-shaped (Fig. 2.6,A). The knife is sharpened by a process known as *honing* and *stropping*. Honing is done manually on a stone or on an electrically operated automatic hone. After honing, stropping is done which is polishing of its edge over a leather strop. The process of sharpening of microtome knife can also be done by automatic knife sharpener (Fig. 2.7). Nowadays, disposable blades for microtomy are also available (Fig. 2.6,B,C).

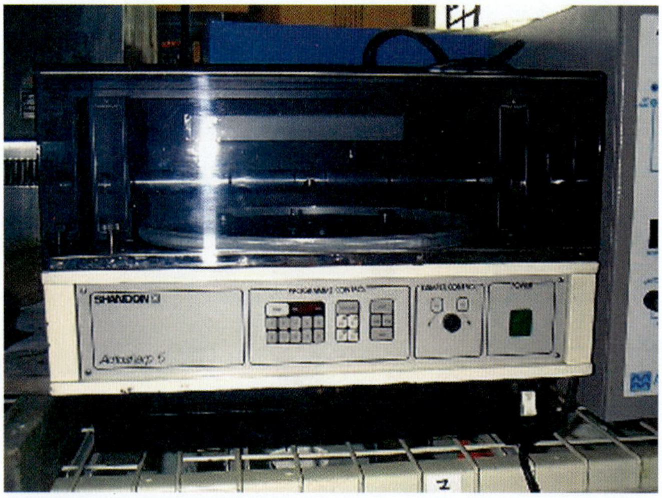

FIGURE 2.7: Automatic knife sharpener, Model Shandon Autosharp 5 (Photograph courtesy of Thermo Shandon, UK through Towa Optics India Pvt. Ltd., Delhi).

2. Sliding Microtome

In this, the tissue block is fixed while the knife is movable. These microtomes are used as freezing microtomes.

3. Freezing Microtome

See under frozen section in Exercise 3.

4. Rocking Microtome

This is a simple microtome. The knife is immovable while the tissue block is held in a spring-bearing rocking arm. It is not used nowadays.

Base-Sledge Microtome

This type of microtome is used for very hard tissues or large blocks e.g. pieces of brain and heart.

Procedure for Microtomy

Put the paraffin block having tissue in it in the rotary microtome. Cut the section by operating the microtome manually after adjusting the thickness at 3-4 μm. Sections are picked from the knife with the help of a forceps or camel hair brush. These are made to float in a tissue floatation bath which is kept at a temperature of 45-50°C i.e. slightly below the melting point of wax (Fig. 2.8). This removes folds in the section. From tissue floatation bath,

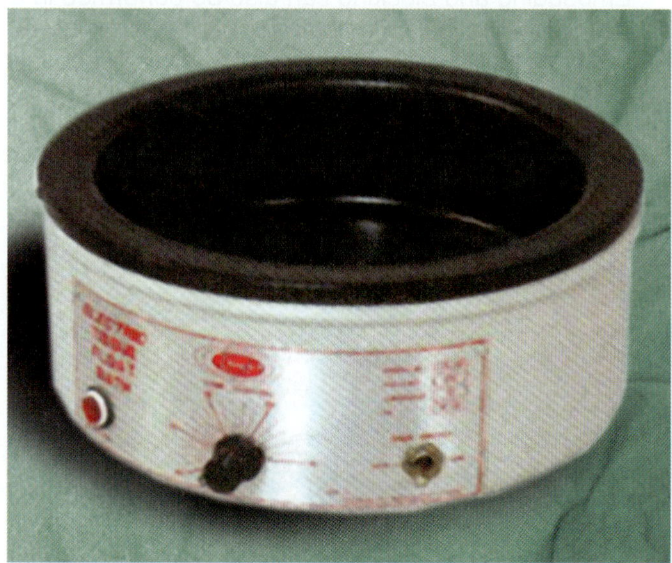

FIGURE 2.8: Tissue floatation bath (Photograph courtesy of Yorco Sales Pvt. Ltd, Delhi).

sections are picked on a clean glass slide. The glass slide is placed in an oven maintained at a temperature of 56°C for 20-30 minutes for proper drying and better adhesion. Coating adhesives for sections can be used before picking up sections; these include egg albumin, gelatin, poly-L-lysine etc. The section is now ready for staining.

ROUTINE STAINING (H & E)

Routine staining is done with haematoxylin and eosin (H & E).

Haematoxylin

This is a natural dye which is obtained from log-wood of tree, *Haematoxylon campechianum.* This tree is commercially grown in Jamaica and Mexico. The natural extract from the stem of this tree is haematoxylin which is an inactive product. This product is oxidised to an active ingredient which is haematein. This process of oxidation is known as *ripening* which can be done naturally in sunlight, or chemically by addition of oxidant like sodium iodate, $KMnO_4$ or mercuric oxide. A *mordant* is added to it (e.g. potash alum) which helps in penetrating the stain particles to the tissue.

Procedure for Staining

Sections are first deparaffinised (removal of wax) by placing the slide in a jar of xylene for 10-15 minutes. As haematoxylin is a water-based dye, the sections before staining are rehydrated which is done by passing the sections in a series of descending grades of alcohol and finally bringing the section to water. Currently, modern laboratories employ automated programmable auto-stainers.

- Place the slide in haematoxylin stain for 8-10 minutes.
- Rinse in water.
- *Differentiation* (i.e. selective removal of excess dye from the section) is done by putting the slide in a solution of 1% acid alcohol for 10 seconds.
- Rinse in water.
- *Blueing* (i.e. bringing of required blue colour to the section) is done by putting the section in Scott's tap water (containing sodium bicarbonate and magnesium sulphate) or saturated solution of lithium carbonate for 2-10 minutes.
- Counterstain with 1% aqueous solution of eosin for 30 seconds to 1 minute.
- One dip in tap water.
- Before mounting, the sections have to be dehydrated which is done by passing the sections in a series of ascending grades of alcohol and finally cleared in xylene, 2-3 dips in each solution.
- Mount in DPX (dextrene polystyrene xylene) or Canada balsam.

Results

Nuclei	:	Blue
Cytoplasm	:	Pink
Muscle, collagen, RBCs, keratin, colloid protein	:	Pink

Exercise 3

Frozen Section and its Staining

Objectives

- Discuss the technique and applications of frozen section.
- Describe the methods of staining for frozen section.

FROZEN SECTION

When a fresh tissue is rapidly frozen, the matter within the tissue turns into ice; in this state the tissue is firm, the ice acting as embedding medium. Therefore, sections are produced without the use of dehydrating solution, clearing agent or wax embedding. This procedure can be carried out in operation theatre complex near the operating table.

Applications

i. It is a rapid intraoperative diagnostic procedure for tissues while the patient is still under anaesthesia.
ii. It is used for determining whether the resection limits of surgical margin are free of tumour or not while the patient is still under anaesthesia.
iii. This is also used for demonstration of some special substances in the cells and tissues e.g. fat, enzymes.

Merits

i. This is a quick diagnostic procedure having a much shorter *turn-around-time* (i.e. time from receipt of tissue to the issue of a final report). The time needed from the receipt of tissue specimen to the study of stained sections is about 10 minutes, while in routine paraffin-sectioning at least two days are required.
ii. Every type of staining can be done.
iii. There is minimal shrinkage of tissues as compared to paraffin sections.
iv. Lipids and enzymes which are lost in routine paraffin sections can be demonstrated.

Demerits

i. It is difficult to cut serial sections.
ii. It is not possible to maintain tissue blocks for future use.
iii. Sections cut are thicker.
iv. Structural details tend to be distorted due to lack of embedding medium.

Methods for Frozen Sections

There are two methods for obtaining frozen sections:

1. Freezing microtome using CO_2 gas
2. Refrigerated microtome (cryostat).

For frozen section, best results are produced from fresh unfixed tissue and freezing the tissue as rapidly as possible.

Freezing Microtome using CO_2 Gas

In this method freezing microtome is used which is a sliding type of microtome.

Setting of microtome and section cutting The microtome is screwed firmly to the edge of a table by means of a stout screw. A CO_2 gas cylinder is placed near the microtome. The cylinder is then connected to the microtome by means of a special tubing. The connecting tube should not have any bends or cracks. Adjust the gauze of the microtome to a required thickness of sections. The knife is inserted in its place. A few drops of water are placed over freezing stage. A selected piece of tissue is placed over stage on drops of water. Short bursts of CO_2 are applied to freeze the tissue and water till the surface of the tissue is completely covered with ice. Alternatively, solid CO_2 (dry ice, cardice) can be used for freezing tissue blocks. Sections are then cut by swinging movement of knife forward and backward with a regular rhythm. The cut sections come over the knife. From the knife, sections are picked with a camel-brush and transferred to a petri dish containing water. The sections are then placed over a glass slide with the help of a dropper. Remove the folds in the sections by tilting the slides. The slide is then passed over flame for a few seconds for fixing the sections over the slide. Section is now ready for staining with a desired stain.

Advantages

i. It is cheap.
ii. It requires less space.
iii. Equipment is portable.

Disadvantages

i. Sections cut are thick.
ii. CO_2 gas may run out in between the procedures.
iii. The connecting tube may be blocked due to solidified CO_2.

Refrigerated Microtome (Cryostat)

In cryostat, a rotary microtome with an antiroll plate housed in a thermostatically-controlled refrigerated cabinet is used. A temperature up to –30°C can be achieved (Fig. 3.1).

Setting of microtome and section cutting Switch on the cryostat along with the knife inserted in position several hours before the procedure for attaining the operating temperature (generally –20°C or lower). A small piece of fresh unfixed tissue (4 mm) is placed on object disc of the deep freeze shelf of the cryostat for 1-2 minutes. The tissue is rapidly frozen. Now the object disc having frozen tissue is inserted into microtome object clamp. Place antiroll plate in its position. By manual movement, sections are cut at desired thickness. The antiroll plate prevents folding of sections. The section is picked from the knife directly on to the clean albuminised glass slide. A glass slide is lowered on to the knife 1 mm from section. The section comes automatically on the glass slide because of difference of temperature between the section and the slide. The section is ready for staining. The cryostat is defrosted and cleaned on weekends.

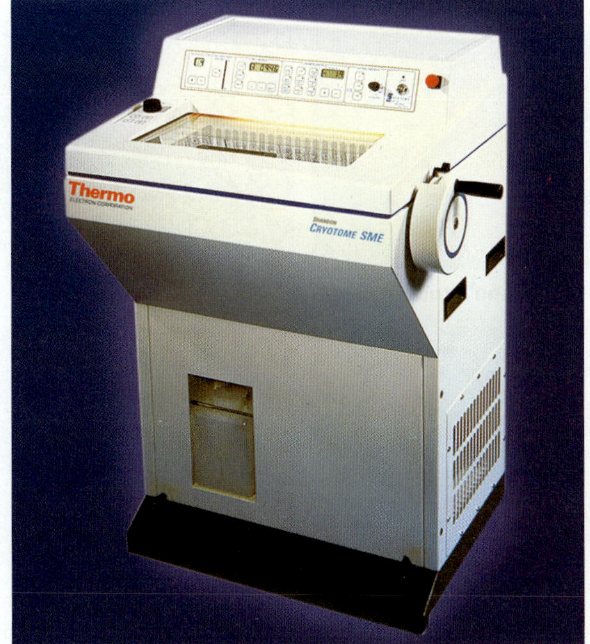

FIGURE 3.1: Cryostat, Model Cryotome (Photograph courtesy of Thermo Shandon, UK through Towa Optics India Pvt. Ltd., Delhi).

Advantages

i. Sections cut are thin.
ii. There is better control of temperature.
iii. Equipment is portable.

Disadvantage

Equipment is expensive.

STAINING OF FROZEN SECTIONS

Sections obtained by freezing microtomy by either of the methods are stained by rapid method as under:

Rapid H & E Staining

- Place the section in haematoxylin for one minute.
- Rinse in tap water.
- Differentiate in 1% acid alcohol by giving one rapid dip.
- Rinse in water.
- Quick blueing is done by passing the section over ammonia vapours or rapid dip in a blueing solution.
- Rinse in tap water.
- Counterstain with 1% aqueous eosin for 3-6 seconds.
- Rinse in tap water.
- Dehydrate by passing the section through 95% alcohol and absolute alcohol, one dip in each solution.
- Clearing is done by passing the section through xylene, one dip.
- Mount in DPX.
- Examine under the microscope.

Toluidine Blue Staining

- Place the section in toluidine blue 0.5% for ½ to 1 minute.
- Rinse in water.
- Mount in water glycerine (i.e. aqueous mountant) with coverslip.
- Examine under the microscope.

Exercise

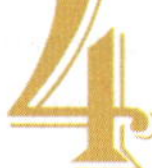

Special Stains and Immunohistochemistry

Objectives

- Describe broad principles and interpretation of results of common special stains.
- Discuss briefly the principle and applications of common immunohistochemical stains.

SPECIAL STAINS

Special stains, also called histochemical stains, are applied for demonstration of certain specific substances/ constituents of the cells/ tissues. The staining depends upon physical, chemical or differential solubility of the stain with the tissues. The principles of some of the staining procedures are well known while those of others are unknown. Some of the common special stains in use in histopathology laboratory are as under (Fig. 4.1):

Sudan Black/Oil Red O

Both these stains are used for demonstration of fat.

Principle Sudan black and Oil red O staining are based on physical combination of the stain with fat. It involves differential solubility of stain in fat because these stains are more soluble in fat than the solvent in which these are prepared. The stain leaves the solvent and goes into the fat.

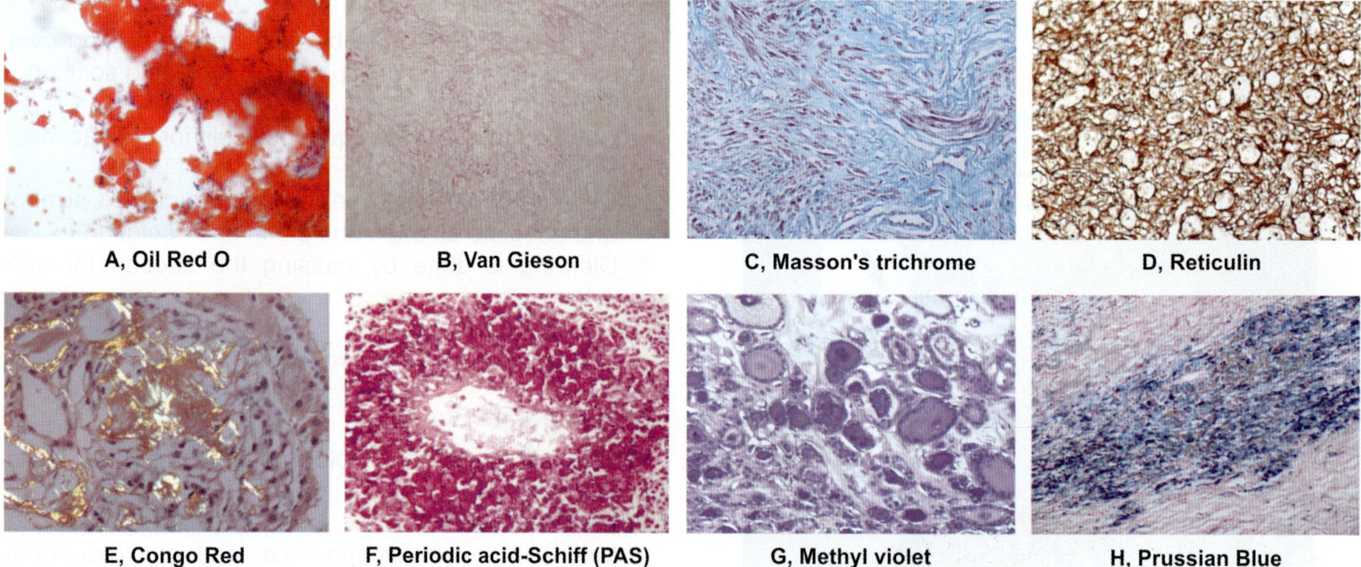

FIGURE 4.1: Common special stains. A, Oil Red O for fat. B, Van Gieson for collagen. C, Masson's trichrome for muscle. D, Reticulin for reticulin fibre. E. Congo Red for amyloid. F, Periodic acid-Schiff (PAS) for glycogen. G, Methyl violet for metachromasia. H, Prussian Blue for iron.

Result

With Oil red O

Fat	:	Bright red
Nuclei	:	Blue

With Sudan black

Fat	:	Black
Nuclei	:	Red

van Gieson

This stain is used for staining of collagen fibres.

Principle It is based on the differential staining of collagen and other tissues (e.g. muscle) depending upon the porosity of tissue and the size of the dye molecule. Collagen with larger pore size takes up the larger molecule red dye (acid fuschin) in an acidic medium, while non-porous muscle stains with much smaller molecule dye (picric acid).

Result

Collagen	:	Red
Nuclei	:	Blue
Other tissues (including muscle)	:	Yellow

Masson's Trichrome

This stain is used for staining of muscle.

Principle Principle is the same as for van Gieson.

Result

Muscle	:	Red
Nuclei	:	Blue-black
Collagen	:	Blue-green

Reticulin

This is used for demonstration of reticulin fibres.

Principle Reticulin stain employs silver impregnation method. There is local reduction and selective precipitation of silver salt.

Result

Reticulin fibres	:	Black
Nuclei	:	Colourless
Collagen	:	Brown

Congo Red

This stain is used for demonstration of amyloid, an extracellular fibrillar proteinaceous substance.

Principle Congo red dye has selective affinity for amyloid and attaches through non-polar hydrogen bonds. It gives green birefringenece when viewed by polarised light.

Result

Amyloid elastic fibres	:	Red

Only amyloid gives green birefringence in polarised light.

Periodic Acid-Schiff (PAS)

This stain is used for demonstration of glycogen and mucopolysaccharides.

Principle Tissues/cells containing 1,2 glycol group are converted into dialdehyde with the help of an oxidising agent which then reacts with Schiff's reagent to give bright magenta colour. Normally Schiff's reagent is colourless.

Result

PAS positive substances	:	Bright pink
Nuclei	:	Blue

PAS positive substances are glycogen, amyloid, colloid, neutral mucin and hyaline cast.

Methyl Violet

This is a metachromatic stain i.e. the tissues are stained in a colour which is different from the colour of the stain itself. It is used for demonstration of amyloid in tissue.

Principle This depends upon the type of dye (stain) used and character of the tissue which unites with the dye. Tissues containing SO_4, PO_4 or COOH groups react with basic dyes and cause their polymerization, which in turn leads to production of colour different from the original dye.

Result

Metachromatic positive tissue	:	Red to violet
Other tissues and background	:	Blue

Other metachromatic stains used are crystal violet, toluidine blue. Metachromatic positive substances are amyloid, mucin and hyaline.

Prussian Blue/Perl's Reaction

This is used for demonstration of iron.

Principle Ferric ions present in the tissue combine with potassium ferrocyanide forming ferric-ferrocyanide.

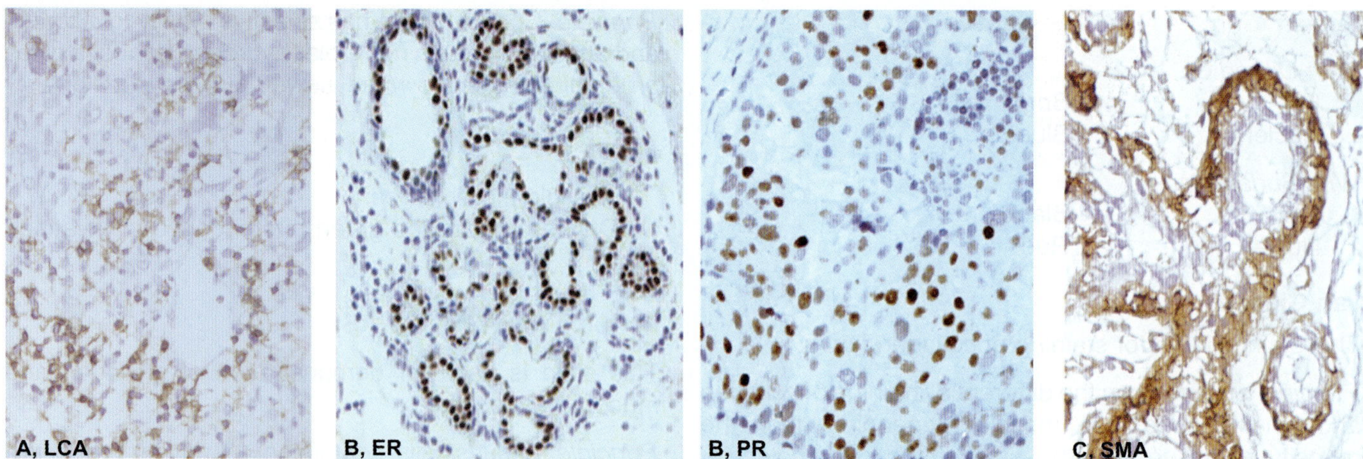

FIGURE 4.2: Examples of IHC stains. A, Membranous staining for LCA. B, Nuclear staining for ER/PR in breast carcinoma. C, Cytoplasmic staining for smooth muscle antigen (SMA) in myoepithelium in breast acinus.

Result

Iron	:	Blue
Cytoplasm and nuclei	:	Red to pink

IMMUNOHISTOCHEMICAL STAINS

Immunohistochemistry (IHC) is the application of immunologic techniques to the cellular pathology.

Principle The technique of IHC is used to detect the status and localisation of particular antigen in the cells (membrane, cytoplasm or nucleus) by use of specific antibodies which are then visualised by chromogen. This then helps in determining cell lineage specifically, or is used to confirm a specific infection.

Technique of IHC

Immunoperoxidase technique employing labelled antibody method to *formalin-fixed paraffin sections* is now widely used. Currently, the two most commonly used procedures in IHC are as under:

i) Peroxidase-antiperoxidase (PAP) method in which PAP reagent, a stable immune-complex, is linked to the primary antibody by a bridging antibody.

ii) Avidin-biotin conjugate (ABC) immunoenzymatic technique in which biotinylated secondary antibody serves to link the primary antibody to a large preformed complex of avidin, biotin and peroxidase.

Interpretation

It is important to remember that *different antigens are localised at different sites in cells* (membrane, cytoplasm or nucleus) and accordingly positive staining is seen and interpreted at those sites e.g. membranous staining for leucocyte common antigen (LCA), nuclear staining for estrogen-progesterone receptors (ER-PR), cytoplasmic staining for smooth muscle actin (SMA) etc (Fig. 4.2).

Applications of IHC

Use of IHC gives objectivity, specificity and reproducibility to the surgical pathologist's diagnosis. IHC stains are used for the following purposes, in order of diagnostic utility:

1. *Tumours of uncertain histogenesis:* A panel of antibodies is chosen to resolve diagnostic problem cases; the selection of antibodies being made is based on clinical history, morphologic features, and results of other relevant investigations.

2. *Prognostic markers in cancer:* These include: proto-oncogenes (e.g. HER-2/neu overexpression in carcinoma breast), tumour suppressor genes or antioncogenes (e.g. *Rb* gene, *p53*), growth factor receptors (e.g. epidermal growth factor receptor or EGFR), and tumour cell proliferation markers (e.g. Ki67, proliferation cell nuclear antigen PCNA).

3. *Prediction of response to therapy:* IHC is widely used to predict therapeutic response in two important tumours—carcinoma of the breast and prostate. The results of oestrogen-receptors and progesterone-receptors in breast cancer have significant prognostic correlation, though the results of androgen-receptor studies in prostatic cancer have limited prognostic value.

4. *Infections:* IHC stains are applied to confirm infectious agent in tissues by use of specific antibodies against microbial DNA or RNA e.g. detection of viruses (HBV, CMV, HPV, herpesviruses), bacteria (e.g. *Helicobacter pylori*), and parasites (*Pneumocystis carinii*) etc.

However, IHC stains cannot be applied to distinguish between neoplastic and non-neoplastic lesions, or between benign and malignant tumours. These distinctions have to be done by traditional methods in surgical pathology.

Section Two

CLINICAL PATHOLOGY AND BASIC CYTOPATHOLOGY

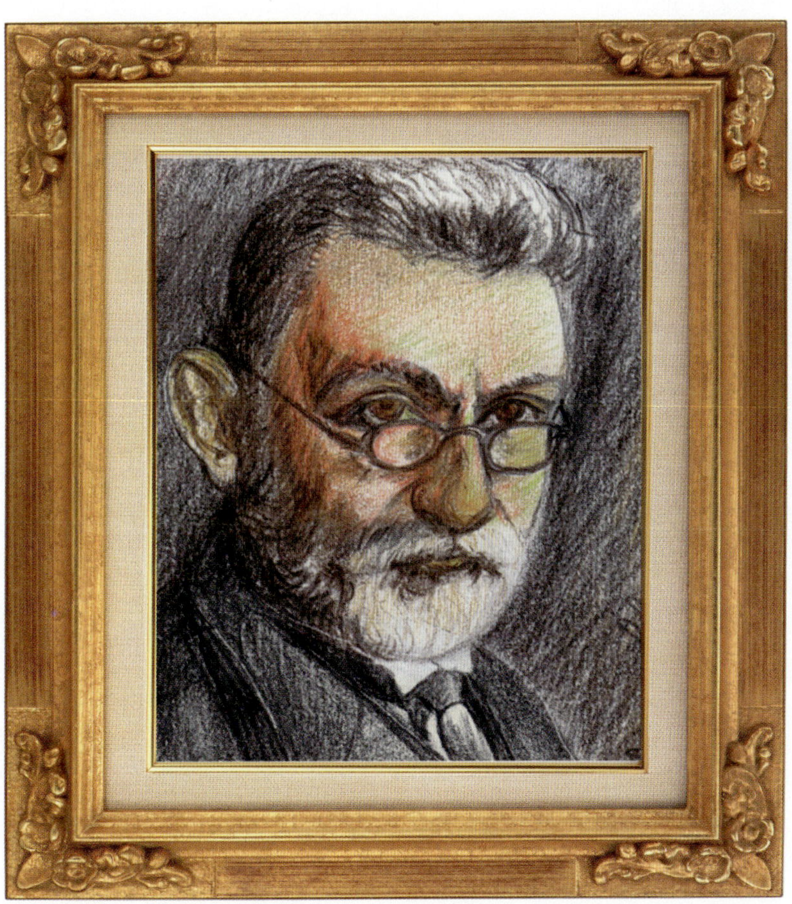

PAUL EHRLICH (1854–1915)
'IMMUNOLOGIST AND CLINICAL PATHOLOGIST'

German Physician, winner of Nobel Prize for his work in immunology; described Ehrlich's test for urobilinogen; staining techniques of cells and bacteria, and laid the foundations of hacmatology.

Section Contents

Exercise

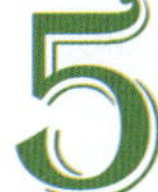

5

Urine Examination I: Physical and Chemical

Objectives

- What are the physical characteristics of normal and abnormal urine?
- Describe the principle, technique and interpretation of various routine tests for chemical constituents of a urinary sample.

Examination of urine is important for diagnosis and assistance in the diagnosis of various diseases. Routine (complete) examination of urine is divided into four parts:

A. Adequacy of specimen
B. Physical/gross examination
C. Chemical examination
D. Microscopic examination

The last named, microscopic examination, is discussed separately in the next exercise.

A. ADEQUACY OF SPECIMEN

The specimen should be properly collected in a clean container which should be properly labelled with name of the patient, age and sex, identity number with date and time of collection. It should not show signs of contamination.

Specimen Collection

For routine examination a clean glass tube or capped jar is used; for bacteriologic examination a sterilized tube or bottle is required. A mid-stream sample is preferable i.e. first part of urine is discarded and mid-stream sample is collected. For 24 hour sample, collection of urine is started in the morning at 8 AM and subsequent samples are collected till next day 8 AM.

Methods of Preservation of Urine

Urine should be examined fresh or within one hour of voiding. But if it has to be delayed then following preservatives can be used which prevent its decomposition:

i. *Refrigeration* at 4°C.
ii. *Toluene:* Toluene is used 1 ml per 50 ml of urine. It acts by forming a surface layer and it preserves the chemical constituents of urine.
iii. *Formalin:* 6-8 drops of 40% formalin per 100 ml of urine is used. It preserves RBCs and pus cells. However, its use has the disadvantage that it gives false-positive test for sugar.
iv. *Thymol:* Thymol is a good preservative; 1% solution of thymol is used. Its use has the disadvantage that it gives false-positive test for proteins.
v. *Acids:* Hydrochloric acid, sulfuric acid and boric acid can also be used as a preservative.

B. PHYSICAL EXAMINATION

Physical examination of urine consists of volume, colour, odour, reaction/pH and specific gravity.

Volume

Normally 700-2500 ml (average 1200 ml) of urine is passed in 24 hours and most of it is passed during day time.

i) Nocturia Nocturia means when urine is passed in excess of 500 ml during night. This is a sign of early renal failure.

ii) Polyuria Polyuria is when excess of urine is passed in 24 hours (> 2500 ml). Polyuria can be physiological due to excess water intake, may be seasonal (e.g. in winter), or can be pathological (e.g. in diabetes insipidus, diabetes mellitus).

iii) Oliguria When less than 500 ml of urine is passed in 24 hours, it is termed as oliguria. It can be due to less intake of water, dehydration, renal ischaemia.

iv) Anuria When there is almost complete suppression of urine (< 150 ml) in 24 hours. It can be due to renal stones, tumours, renal ischaemia.

Colour

Normally urine is clear, pale or straw-coloured due to pigment urochrome.

i) Colourless in diabetes mellitus, diabetes insipidus, excess intake of water.

ii) Deep amber colour due to good muscular exercise, high grade fever.

iii) Orange colour due to increased urobilinogen, concentrated urine.

iv) Smoky urine due to small amount of blood, administration of vitamin B_{12}, aniline dye.

v) Red due to haematuria, haemoglobinuria.

vi) Brown due to bile.

vii) Milky due to pus, fat.

viii) Green due to putrefied sample, phenol poisoning.

Odour

Normally urine has faint aromatic odour.

i) Pungent due to ammonia produced by bacterial contamination.

ii) Putrid due to UTI.

iii) Fruity due to ketoacidosis.

iv) Mousy due to phenylketonuria.

Reaction/pH

It reflects ability of the kidney to maintain H^+ ion concentration in extracellular fluid and plasma. It can be measured by pH indicator paper or by electronic pH meter.

Freshly voided normal urine is slightly acidic and its pH ranges from 4.6-7.0 (average 6.0).

- *Acidic urine* is due to the following:
  - i. High protein intake, e.g. meat.
  - ii. Ingestion of acidic fruits.
  - iii. Respiratory and metabolic acidosis.
  - iv. UTI by *E. coli.*
- *Alkaline urine* is due to following:
  - i. Citrus fruits.
  - ii. Vegetables.
  - iii. Respiratory and metabolic alkalosis.
  - iv. UTI by *Proteus, Pseudomonas.*

Specific Gravity

This is the ratio of weight of 1 ml volume of urine to that of weight of 1 ml of distilled water. It depends upon the concentration of various particles/solutes in the urine. Specific gravity is used to measure the concentrating and diluting power of the kidneys. It can be measured by urinometer, refractometer or reagent strips.

1. Urinometer

Procedure

- Fill urinometer container 3/4th with urine.
- Insert urinometer into it so that it floats in urine without touching the wall and bottom of container (Fig. 5.1).
- Read the graduation on the arm of urinometer at lower urinary meniscus.
- Add or substract 0.001 from the final reading for each 3°C above or below the calibration temperature respectively marked on the urinometer.

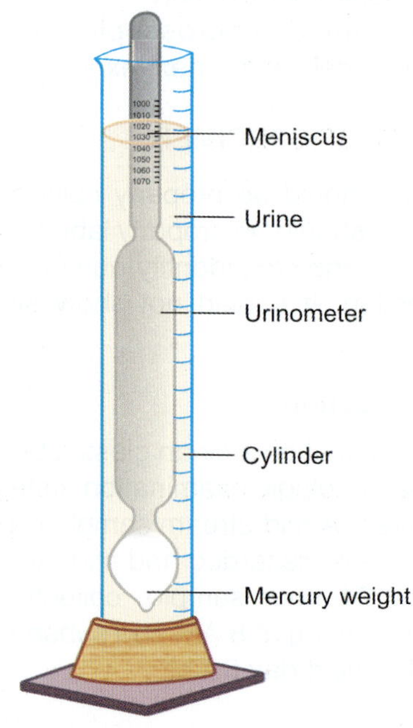

FIGURE 5.1: Urinometer and the container for floating it for measuring specific gravity.

2. Refractometer

It measures the refractive index of urine. This procedure requires only a few drops of urine in contrast to urinometer where approximately 100 ml of urine is required.

3. Reagent Strip Method

This method employs the use of chemical reagent strip (see Fig. 5.3, page 22).

Significance of Specific Gravity

The normal specific gravity of urine is 1.003 to 1.030.

Low specific gravity urine occurs in:

i. Excess water intake
ii. Diabetes insipidus

High specific gravity urine is seen in:

i. Dehydration
ii. Albuminuria
iii. Glycosuria

Fixed specific gravity (1.010) of urine is seen in:

i. ADH deficiency
ii. Chronic nephritis

C. CHEMICAL EXAMINATION

Chemical constituents frequently tested in urine are: proteins, glucose, ketones, bile derivatives and blood.

Tests for Proteinuria

If urine is not clear, it should be filtered or centrifuged before testing. Urine may be tested for proteinuria by qualitative tests and quantitative methods.

Qualitative Tests for Proteinuria

1. Heat and acetic acid test
2. Sulfosalicylic acid test
3. Heller's test
4. Reagent strip method.

1. Heat and Acetic Acid Test

Heat causes coagulation of proteins. The procedure is as under:

- Take a 5 ml test tube.
- Fill 2/3rd with urine.
- Acidify by adding a few drops of 3% glacial acetic acid if urine is alkaline.
- Boil upper portion for 2 minutes (lower part acts as control).

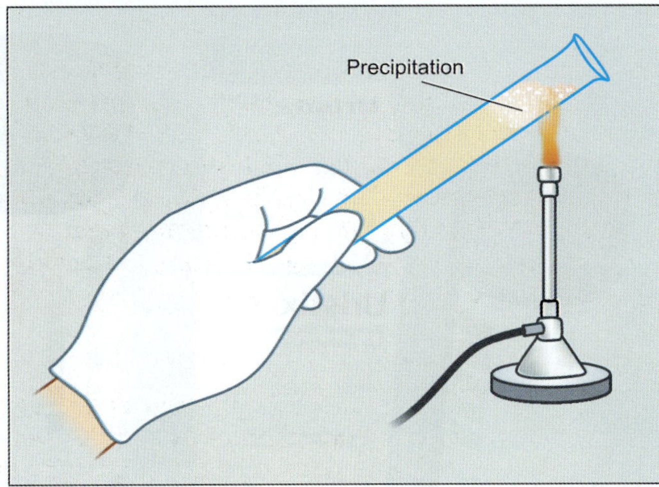

FIGURE 5.2: Heat and acetic acid test for proteinuria. Note the method of holding the tube from the bottom while heating the upper part.

- If precipitation or turbidity appears, add a few drops of 10% acetic acid.

Interpretation If turbidity or precipitation disappears on addition of acetic acid, it is due to phosphates; if it persists after addition of acetic acid, then it is due to proteins. Depending upon amount of protein, the results are interpreted as under (Fig. 5.2):

No cloudiness	=	negative.
Faint cloudiness	=	traces (less than 0.1 g/dl).
Cloudiness without granularity	=	+(0.1 g/dl).
Granular cloudiness	=	++(0.1-0.2 g/dl)
Precipitation and flocculation	=	+++(0.2-0.4 g/dl).
Thick solid precipitation	=	++++ (0.5 g/dl).

2. Sulfosalicylic Acid Test

This is a very reliable test. The procedure is as under:

- Make urine acidic by adding acetic acid.
- To 2 ml of urine add a few drops (4-5) of 20% sulfosalicylic acid.

Interpretation Appearance of turbidity which persists after heating indicates presence of proteins.

3. Heller's Test

- Take 2 ml of concentrated nitric acid in a test tube.
- Add urine drop by drop by the side of test tube.

Interpretation Appearance of white ring at the junction indicates presence of protein.

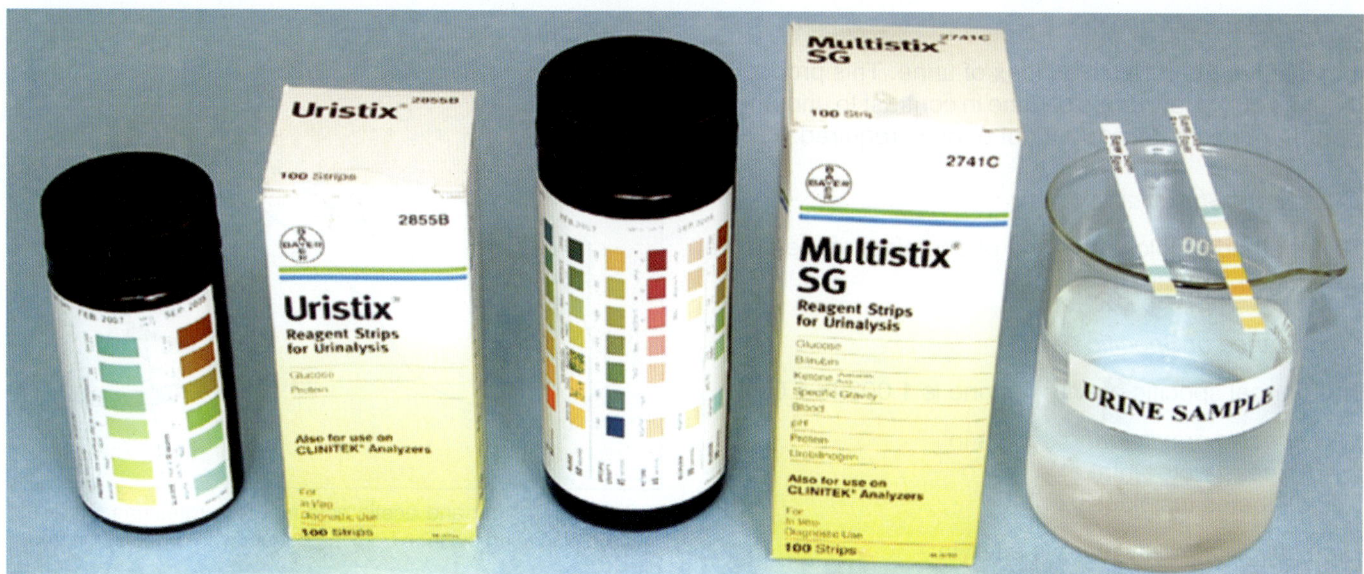

FIGURE 5.3: Strip method for testing various constituents in urine. Multistix 10 SG, and Uristix (Photograph courtesy of Bayer Diagnostics, Baroda, India).

4. *Reagent Strip Method*

Bromophenol coated strip is dipped in urine. Change in colour of strip indicates presence of proteins in urine and is compared with the colour chart provided for semiquantitative grading (Fig. 5.3).

Quantitative Estimation of Proteins in Urine

1. Esbach's albuminometer method
2. Turbidimetric method.

1. *Esbach's albuminometer method*

- Fill the albuminometer with urine upto mark U.
- Add Esbach's reagent (picric acid + citric acid) upto mark R (Fig. 5.4).
- Stopper the tube, mix it and let it stand for 24 hours.
- Take the reading from the level of precipitation in the albuminometer tube and divide it by 10 to get the percentage of proteins.

2. *Turbidimetric method*

- Take 1 ml of urine and 1 ml standard in two separate tubes.
- Add 4 ml of trichloroacetic acid to each tube.
- After 5 minutes take the reading with red filter (680 nm).

Causes of Proteinuria

Normally, there is a very scanty amount of protein in urine (< 150 mg/day).

- *Heavy proteinuria* (> 3 gm/day) occurs due to:
  - i. Nephrotic syndrome
  - ii. Renal vein thrombosis
  - iii. Diabetes mellitus
  - iv. SLE

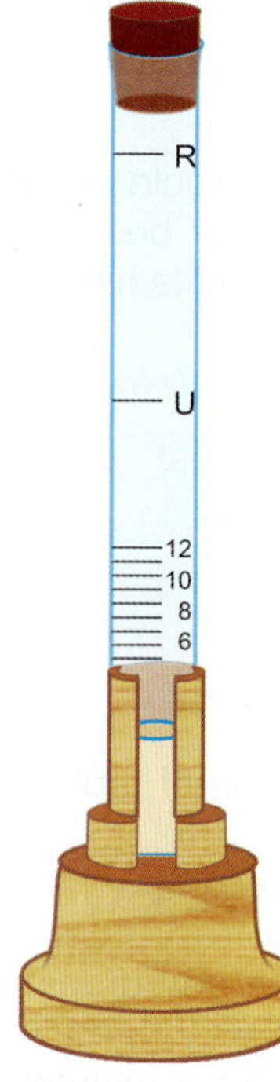

FIGURE 5.4: Esbach's albuminometer for quantitative estimation of proteins (U = urine; R = Esbach's reagent).

- *Moderate proteinuria* (1-3 gm/day) is seen in:
  i. Chronic glomerulonephritis
  ii. Nephrosclerosis
  iii. Multiple myeloma
  iv. Pyelonephritis
- *Mild proteinuria* (< 1.0 gm/day) occurs in:
  i. Hypertension
  ii. Polycystic kidney
  iii. Chronic pyelonephritis
  iv. UTI
  v. Fever.
- *Microalbuminuria* is excretion of albumin 30-300 mg/day or random urine albumin/creatinine ratio of 30-300 mg/gm creatinine and is indicative of early and possibly reversible glomerular damage from hypertension and risk factor for cardiovascular disease. *Microalbuminuria* is estimated by radioimmunoassay.

Test for Bence Jones Proteinuria

Bence Jones proteins are light chains of γ-globulin. These are excreted in multiple myeloma and other paraproteinaemias. In heat and acetic acid test performed under temperature control, these proteins are precipitated at lower temperature (56°C) and disappear on further heating above 90°C but reappear on cooling to lower temperature again. In case both albumin as well as Bence Jones proteins are present in urine, the sample of urine is heated to boiling. Precipitates so formed due to albumin are filtered out and the test for Bence Jones proteins is repeated under temperature control as above.

Test for Glucosuria

Glucose is by far the most important of the sugars which may appear in urine. Normally approximately 130 mg of glucose per 24 hours is passed in urine which is undetectable by qualitative tests.

Tests for glucosuria may be qualitative or quantitative.

Qualitative Tests

These are as under:
1. Benedict's test
2. Reagent strip test

1. Benedict's Test

In this test cupric ion is reduced by glucose to cuprous oxide and a coloured precipitate is formed.

Procedure
- Take 5 ml of Benedict's qualitative reagent in a test tube.
- Add 8 drops (or 0.5 ml) of urine.
- Heat to boiling for 2 minutes (Fig. 5.5).
- Cool in water bath or in running tap water and look for colour change and precipitation.

Interpretation

No change of blue colour	=	Negative
Greenish colour	=	traces (< 0.5 g/dl)
Green/cloudy green ppt	=	+ (0.5-1 g/dl)
Yellow ppt	=	++ (1-1.5 g/dl)
Orange ppt	=	+++ (1.5-2 g/dl)
Brick red ppt	=	++++ (> 2 g/dl)

Since Benedict's test is for reducing substances excreted in the urine, the test is positive for all reducing

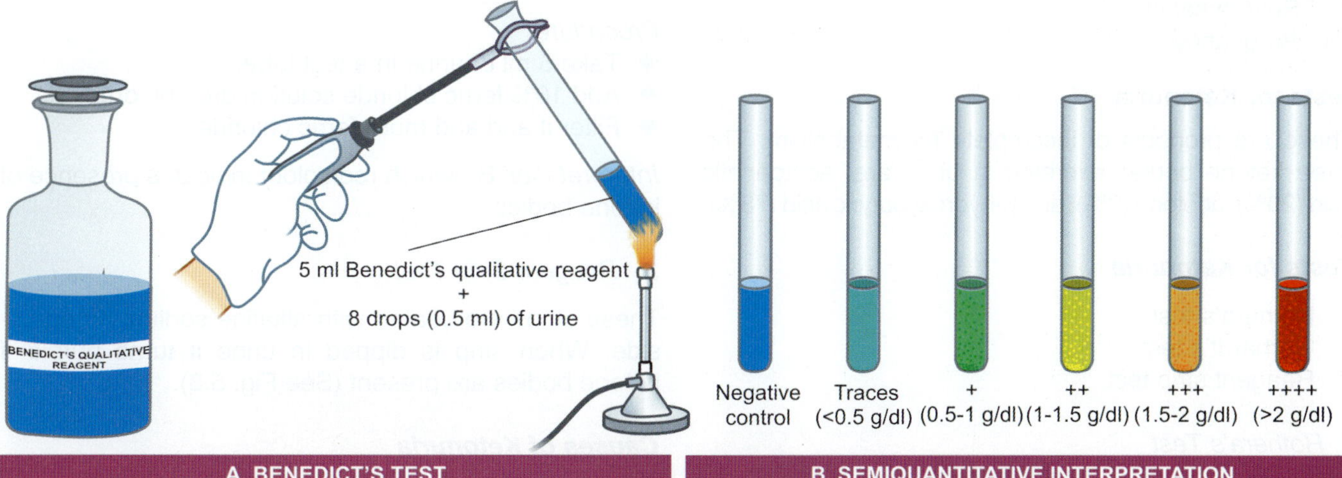

FIGURE 5.5: A, Method for Benedict's test (qualitative) for glucosuria. The test sample shows brick red precipitation (++++). B, Semiquantitative interpretation of glucosuria by Benedict's test.

sugars (glucose, fructose, maltose, lactose *but not for sucrose which is a non-reducing sugar*) and other reducing substances (e.g. ascorbic acid, salicylates, antibiotics, L-dopa).

2. Reagent Strip Test

These strips are coated with glucose oxidase and the test is based on enzymatic reaction. This test is specific for glucose. The strip is dipped in urine for 10 seconds. If there is change in colour of strip it indicates presence of glucose. The colour change is matched with standard colour chart provided on the label of the reagent strip bottle (see Fig. 5.3).

Quantitative Test for Glucose

Procedure Take 25 ml of quantitative Benedict's reagent in a conical flask. Add to it 15 gm of sodium carbonate (crystalline) and some pieces of porcelain and heat it to boil. Add urine to it from a burette slowly till there is disappearance of blue colour of Benedict's reagent. Note the volume of urine used. Calculate the amount of glucose present in urine as under:

$$\frac{0.05 \times 100}{\text{Amount of urine}}$$

(0.05 gm of glucose reduces 25 ml of Benedict's reagent).

Causes of Glucosuria

i. Diabetes mellitus
ii. Renal glucosuria
iii. Severe burns
iv. Administration of corticosteroids
v. Severe sepsis
vi. Pregnancy

Tests for Ketonuria

These are products of incomplete fat metabolism. The three ketone bodies excreted in urine are: acetoacetic acid (20%), acetone (2%), and β-hydroxybutyric acid (78%).

Tests for Ketonuria

1. Rothera's test
2. Gerhardt's test
3. Reagent strip test

1. Rothera's Test

Principle Ketone bodies (acetone and acetoacetic acid) combine with alkaline solution of sodium nitroprusside forming purple complex.

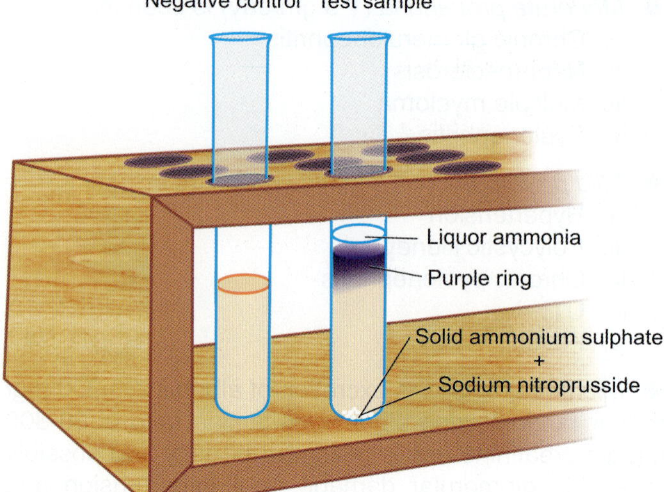

FIGURE 5.6: Rothera's test for ketone bodies in urine showing purple coloured ring in positive test.

Procedure

- Take 5 ml of urine in a test tube.
- Saturate it with solid ammonium sulphate salt; it will start sedimenting to the bottom of the tube when saturated.
- Add a few crystals of sodium nitroprusside and shake.
- Add liquor ammonia from the side of test tube.

Interpretation Appearance of purple or permangnate coloured ring at the junction indicates presence of ketone bodies (Fig. 5.6).

2. Gerhardt's Test

It is not a very sensitive test.

Procedure

- Take 5 ml of urine in a test tube.
- Add 10% ferric chloride solution drop by drop.
- Filter it and add more ferric chloride.

Interpretation Brownish red colour indicates presence of ketone bodies.

3. Reagent Strip Test

These strips are coated with alkaline sodium nitroprusside. When strip is dipped in urine it turns purple if ketone bodies are present (See Fig. 5.3).

Causes of Ketonuria

i. Diabetic ketoacidosis
ii. Dehydration
iii. Hyperemesis gravidarum

iv. Fever
v. Cachexia
vi. After general anaesthesia

Test for Bile Derivatives in Urine

Three bile derivatives excreted in urine are: urobilinogen, bile salts and bile pigments. While urobilinogen is normally excreted in urine in small amounts, bile salts and bile pigments appear in urine in liver diseases only.

Tests for Bile Salts

Bile salts excreted in urine are cholic acid and chenodeoxycholic acid. Tests for bile salts are Hay's test and strip method.

1. Hay's Test

Principle Bile salts if present in urine lower the surface tension of the urine.

Procedure
- Fill a 50 or 100 ml beaker 2/3rd to 3/4th with urine.
- Sprinkle finely powdered sulphur powder over it (Fig. 5.7).

Interpretation If bile salts are present in the urine then sulphur powder sinks, otherwise it floats.

2. Strip Method

Coated strips can be used for detecting bile salts as for other constituents in urine (see Fig. 5.3).

Cause for bile salts in urine
i. Obstructive jaundice

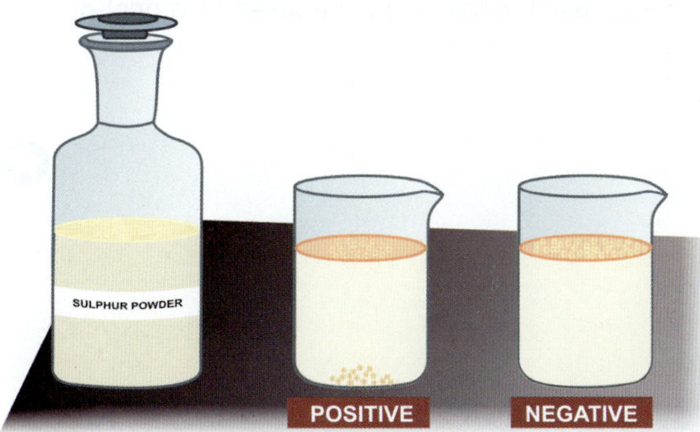

FIGURE 5.7: Hay's test for bile salts in urine. The test is positive in beaker in the centre contrasted with negative control in beaker on right side.

Tests for Urobilinogen

Normally a small amount of urobilinogen is excreted in urine (4 mg/24 hr). The sample should always be collected in a dark coloured bottle as urobilinogen gets oxidised on exposure to light.

Tests for urobilinogen in urine are Ehrlich's test and reagent strip test.

1. Ehrlich's Test

Principle Urobilinogen in urine combines with Ehrlich's aldehyde reagent to give a red purple coloured compound.

Procedure
- Take 10 ml of urine in a test tube.
- Add 1 ml of Ehrlich's aldehyde reagent.
- Wait for 3-5 minutes.

Interpretation Development of red purple colour indicates presence of urobilinogen. A positive test is subsequently done in dilutions; normally it is positive in upto 1:20 dilution.

2. Reagent Strip Test

These strips are coated with p-dimethyl-amino-benz-aldehyde. When strip is dipped in urine, it turns reddish-brown if urobilinogen is present (see Fig. 5.3).

Significance

Causes of increased urobilinogen in urine
i. Haemolytic jaundice and haemolytic anaemia

Causes for absent urobilinogen in urine
ii. Obstructive jaundice

Tests for Bilirubin (Bile Pigment) in Urine

Bilirubin is breakdown product of haemoglobin. Normally no bilirubin is passed in urine.

Following tests are done for detection of bilirubin in urine:
1. Fouchet's test
2. Foam test
3. Reagent strip test

1. Fouchet's Test

Principle Ferric chloride oxidises bilirubin to green biliverdin.

Procedure
- Take 10 ml of urine in a test tube.
- Add 3-5 ml of 10% barium chloride.
- Filter through filter paper.

- To the precipitate on filter paper, add a few drops of Fouchet's reagent (ferric chloride + trichloroacetic acid).

Interpretation Development of green colour indicates bilirubin.

2. Foam Test

It is a non-specific test.

Procedure
- Take 5/10 ml of urine in a test tube.
- Shake it vigorously.

Interpretation Presence of yellow foam at the top indicates presence of bilirubin.

3. Reagent Strip Test

Principle It is based on coupling reaction of bilirubin with diazonium salt with which strip is coated. Dip the strip in urine; if it changes to blue colour then bilirubin is present (see Fig. 5.3).

Causes of bilirubinuria
i) Obstructive jaundice
ii) Hepatocellular jaundice

Tests for Blood in Urine

Tests for detection of blood in urine are as under:
1. Benzidine test
2. Orthotoluidine test
3. Reagent strip test

1. Benzidine Test

Procedure
- Take 2 ml of urine in a test tube.
- Add 2 ml of saturated solution of benzidine with glacial acetic acid.
- Add 1 ml of H_2O_2 to it.

Interpretation Appearance of blue colour indicates presence of blood. Benzidine is, however, carcinogenic and this test is not commonly used.

2. Orthotoluidine Test

Procedure
- Take 2 ml of urine in a test tube.
- Add a solution of 1 ml of orthotoluidine in glacial acetic acid.
- Add a few drops of H_2O_2.

Interpretation Blue or green colour indicates presence of blood in urine.

3. Reagent Strip Test

The reagent strip is coated with orthotoluidine. Dip the strip in urine. If it changes to blue colour then blood is present (see Fig. 5.3).

Causes of blood in urine
i. Renal stones
ii. Renal tumours
iii. Polycystic kidney
iv. Bleeding disorders
v. Trauma.

AUTOMATED URINALYSIS

Currently, fully automated urine chemistry reagent strip analysers are available which are equipped to perform automatic pipetting or test strip dipping, as well as carry out photometric measurement of reagent strip fields. The end result readings can be taken as a print-out.

Exercise

6

Urine Examination II: Microscopy

Objectives

- How is the wet preparation for microscopic examination of urine made and examined?
- Discuss various formed elements seen in the sediment of urine in routine microscopic examination.

Microscopic examination of urine is discussed under four headings:

A. Collection of sample
B. Preparation of sediment
C. Examination of sediment
D. Automation in urine analysis

A. COLLECTION OF SAMPLE

Early morning sample is the best specimen. It provides an acidic and concentrated sample which preserves the formed elements (RBCs, WBCs and casts) which otherwise tend to lyse in a hypotonic or alkaline urine. The specimen should be examined fresh or within 1-2 hours of collection. But if some delay is anticipated, the sample should be preserved as described in the preceding exercise.

B. PREPARATION OF SEDIMENT

- Take 5-10 ml of urine in a centrifuge tube.
- Centrifuge for 5 minutes at 3000 rpm.
- Discard the supernatant.
- Resuspend the deposit in a few ml of urine left.
- Place a drop of this on a clean glass slide.
- Place a coverslip over it and examine it under the microscope.

C. EXAMINATION OF SEDIMENT

Urine is an unstained preparation and its microscopic examination is routinely done under reduced light using the light microscope. This is done by keeping the condenser low with partial closure of diaphragm. First examine it under low power objective, then under high power and keep on changing the fine adjustment in order to visualise the sediments in different planes and report as *number of cells/HPF* (high power field). Phase contrast microscopy may be used for more transluscent formed elements. Rarely, polarising microscopy is used to distinguish crystals and fibres from cellular or protein casts.

Following categories of constituents are frequently reported in the urine on microscopic examination:

1. Cells (RBCs,WBCs, epithelial cells)
2. Casts
3. Crystals
4. Miscellaneous structures

1. Cells in Urine

RBCs

These appear as pale or yellowish, biconcave, double-contoured, disc-like structures, and when viewed from side they have an hour-glass appearance. In hypotonic urine, RBCs swell up while in hypertonic urine they are crenated. They can be confused with WBCs, yeast and air bubbles/oil droplets but can be distinguished as under (Fig. 6.1):

i. The WBCs are larger in size and are granular.
ii. Yeast cells appear round but show budding.

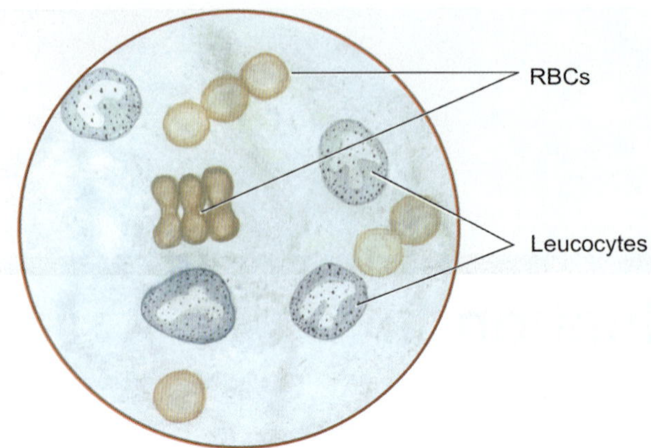

FIGURE 6.1: RBCs and WBCs in the urine sediment.

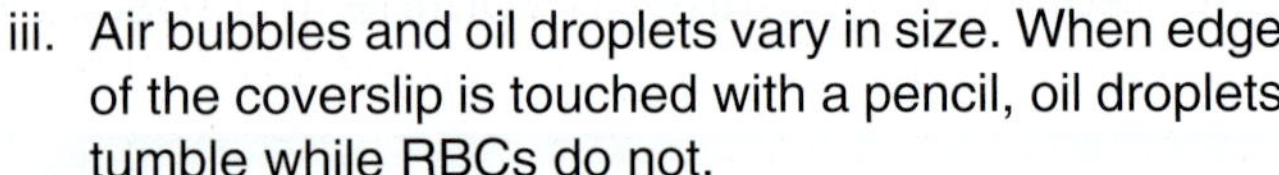

iii. Air bubbles and oil droplets vary in size. When edge of the coverslip is touched with a pencil, oil droplets tumble while RBCs do not.

Significance Normally 0-2 RBCs/HPF may be passed in urine. RBCs in excess of this number are seen in urine in the following conditions:

Physiological

i. Following severe exercise
ii. Smoking
iii. Lumbar lordosis

Pathological

i. Renal stones
ii. Kidney tumours
iii. Glomerulonephritis
iv. Polycystic kidney
v. UTI
vi. Trauma

WBCs

These appear as round granular 12-14 µm in diameter. In fresh urine nuclear details are well visualised (Fig. 6.1). WBCs can be confused with RBCs. For differentiating, add a drop of dilute acetic acid under coverslip. RBCs are lysed while nuclear details of WBCs become more clear. WBCs can also be stained by adding a drop of crystal violet or safranin stain.

Significance Normally 0-4 WBCs/HPF may be present in females. WBCs are seen in urine in following conditions:

Pathological

i. UTI
ii. Cystitis
iii. Prostatitis

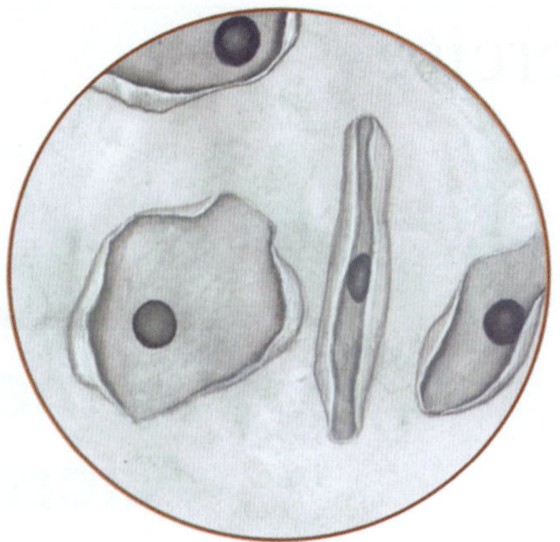

FIGURE 6.2: Squamous epithelial cells in urine, frequently seen in females.

iv. Chronic pyelonephritis
v. Renal stones
vi. Renal tumours

Epithelial Cells

These are round to polygonal cells with a round to oval, small to large nucleus. Epithelial cells in urine can be squamous epithelial cells, tubular cells and transitional cells i.e. they can be from lower or upper urinary tract, and sometime it is difficult to distinguish between different types of these cells. At times, these cells can be confused with cancer cells.

Significance Normally a few epithelial cells are seen in normal urine, more common in females and reflect normal sloughing of these cells (Fig. 6.2).

When these cells are present in large number along with WBCs, they are indicative of inflammation.

2. Casts in Urine

These are formed due to moulding in renal tubules of solidified proteins. Their shape depends upon their site of origin. In general, casts are cylindrical in shape with rounded ends. The basic composition of casts is Tamm-Horsfall protein which is secreted by tubular cells. Casts appear in urine only in renal diseases.

Depending upon the content, casts are of following types (Fig. 6.3):

i. Hyaline cast
ii. Red cell cast
iii. Leucocyte cast
iv. Granular cast
v. Waxy cast
vi. Fatty cast

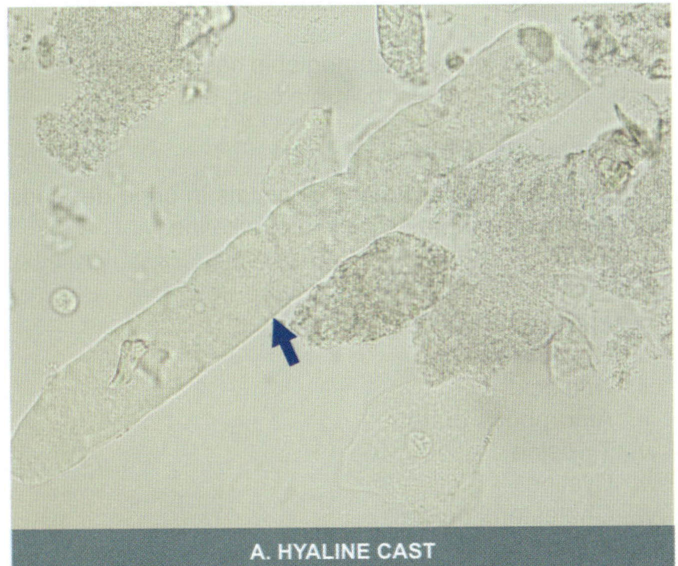

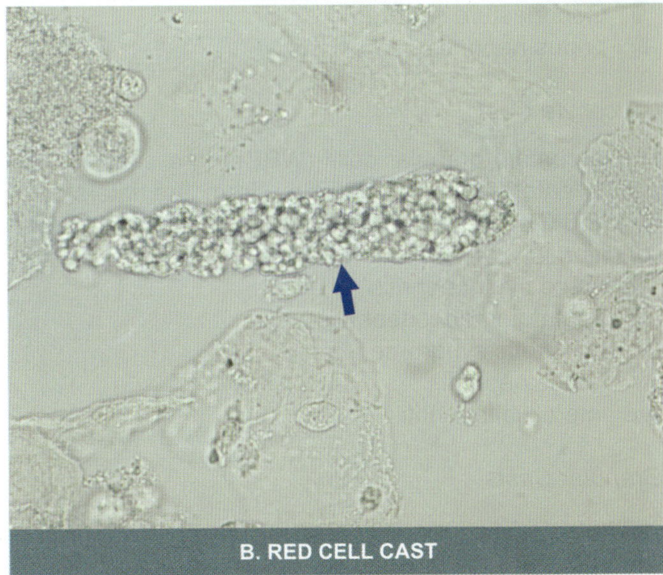

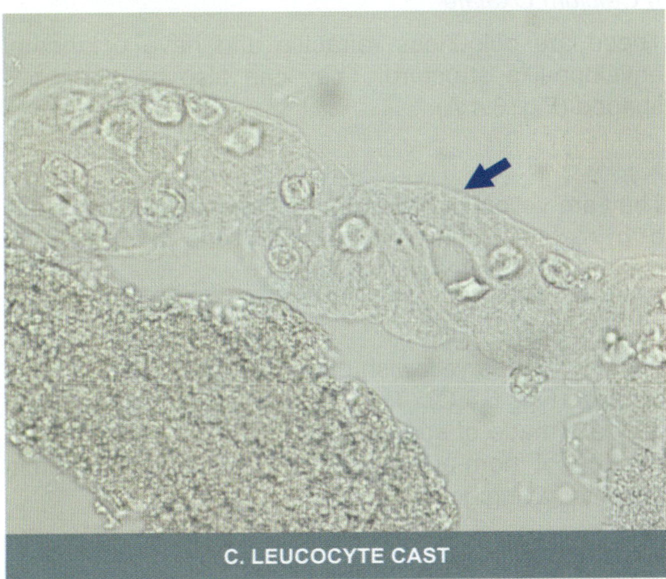

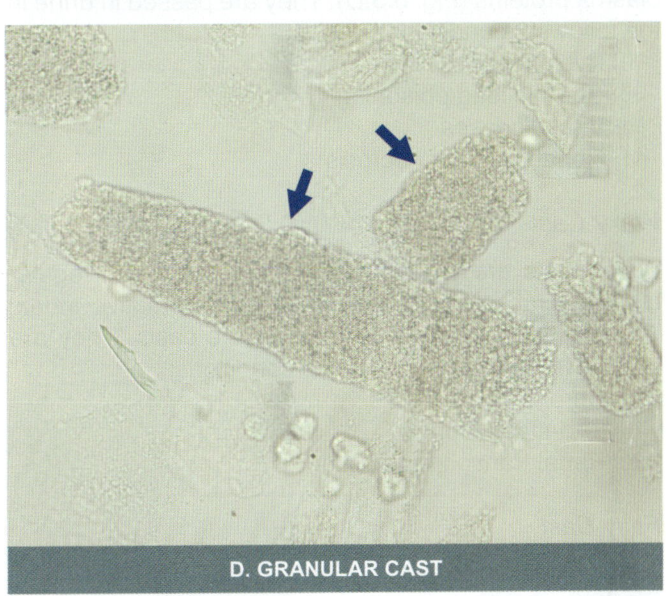

FIGURE 6.3: Various types of casts in urine.

vii. Epithelial cast
viii. Pigment cast

Hyaline Cast

Hyaline cast is basic protein cast. These are cylindrical, colourless homogeneous and transparent (Fig. 6.3,A). They are passed in urine in the following conditions:

i. Fever
ii. Exercise
iii. Acute glomerulonephritis
iv. Malignant hypertension
v. Chronic renal disease

Red Cell Cast

These casts contain RBCs and have a yellowish-orange colour (Fig. 6.3,B). Glomerular damage results in appearance of RBCs into tubules. They are passed in urine in the following conditions:

i. Acute glomerulonephritis
ii. Renal infarct

iii. Goodpasture syndrome
iv. Lupus nephritis

Leucocyte Cast

These contain granular cells (WBCs) in a clear matrix. WBCs enter the tubular lumina from the interstitium (Fig. 6.3,C). They are passed in urine in the following conditions:
i. Acute pyelonephritis
ii. Acute glomerulonephritis
iii. Nephrotic syndrome
iv. Lupus nephritis
v. Interstitial nephritis

Granular Casts

Granular casts have coarse granules in basic matrix. Granules form from degenerating cells or solidification of plasma proteins (Fig. 6.3,D). They are passed in urine in the following conditions:
i. Pyelonephritis
ii. Chronic lead poisoning
iii. Viral diseases
iv. Renal papillary necrosis

Waxy Casts

Waxy casts are yellowish homogeneous with irregular blunt or cracked ends and have high refractive index. These are also known as renal failure casts. They are passed in urine in the following conditions:
i. Chronic renal failure
ii. End-stage kidney
iii. Renal transplant rejection

Fatty Cast

They contain fat globules of varying size which are highly refractile. Fat in the cast is cholesterol or triglycerides. These are passed in urine in the following conditions:
i. Nephrotic syndrome
ii. Fat necrosis

Epithelial Cast

Epithelial casts contain shed off tubular epithelial cells and appear as two parallel rows of cells. Sometimes these are difficult to differentiate from WBC casts. They are passed in urine in following conditions:
i. Acute tubular necrosis
ii. Heavy metal poisoning
iii. Renal transplant rejection

Pigment Cast

Pigment casts include haemoglobin casts, haemosiderin casts, myoglobin casts, bilirubin cast, etc.

3. Crystals in Urine

Formation and appearance of crystals in urine depends upon pH of the urine, i.e. acidic or alkaline.

Crystals in Acidic Urine

These are as under (Fig. 6.4):
i. Calcium oxalate
ii. Uric acid
iii. Amorphous urate
iv. Tyrosine
v. Cystine
vi. Cholesterol crystals
vii. Sulphonamide

i) Calcium Oxalate

These are colourless refractile and have octahedral envelope-like structure. They can also be dumb-bell shaped (Fig. 6.4,A).

ii) Uric Acid

They are yellow or brown rhomboid-shaped seen singly or in rosettes. They can also be in the form of prism, plates and sheaves (Fig. 6.4,B).

iii) Amorphous Urate

They appear as yellowish brown granules in the form of clumps (Fig. 6.4,C). They dissolve on heating. When they are made of sodium urate, they are needle-like in the form of thorn-apple. They are passed more often in patients having gout.

iv) Tyrosine

They are yellowish in the form of silky needles or sheaves (Fig. 6.4,D). They are passed in urine in jaundice.

v) Cystine

They are colourless, hexagonal plates which are highly refractile (Fig. 6.4,E). They are passed in urine in an inborn error of metabolism, cystinuria.

vi) Cholesterol Crystals

These are rare and are seen in urinary tract infection, rupture of lymphatic into renal pelvis or due to blockage of lymphatics (Fig. 6.4,F).

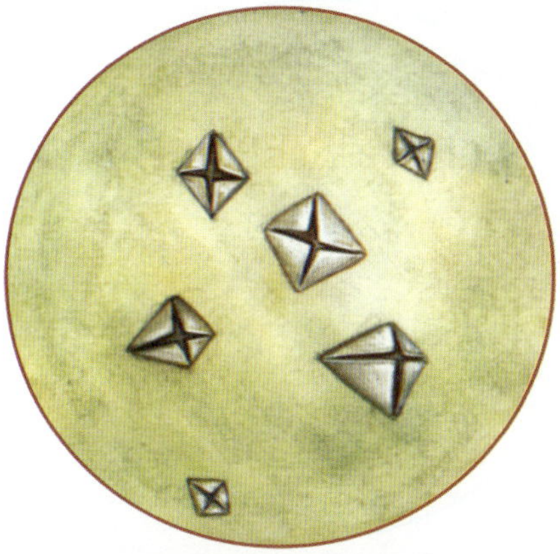

A, CALCIUM OXALATE

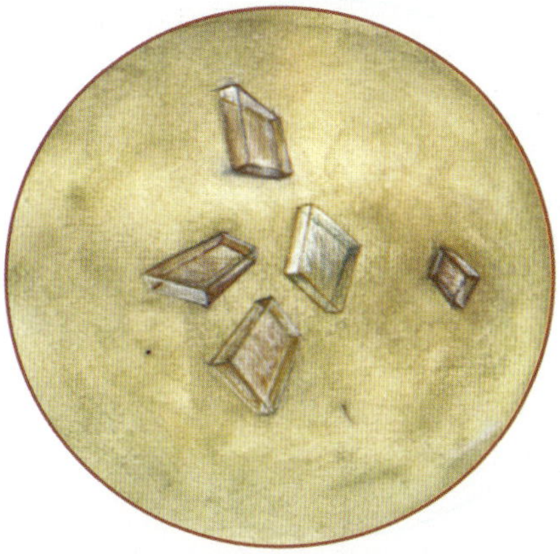

B, URIC ACID

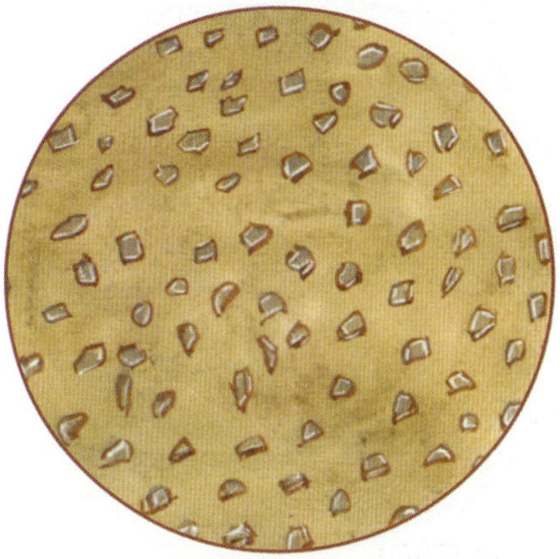

C, AMORPHOUS URATES

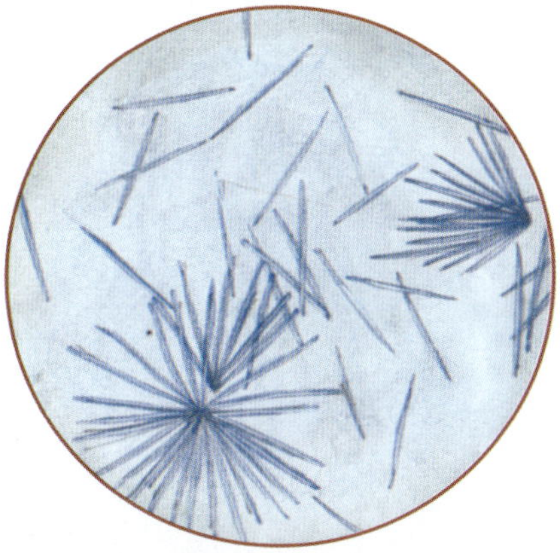

D, TYROSINE

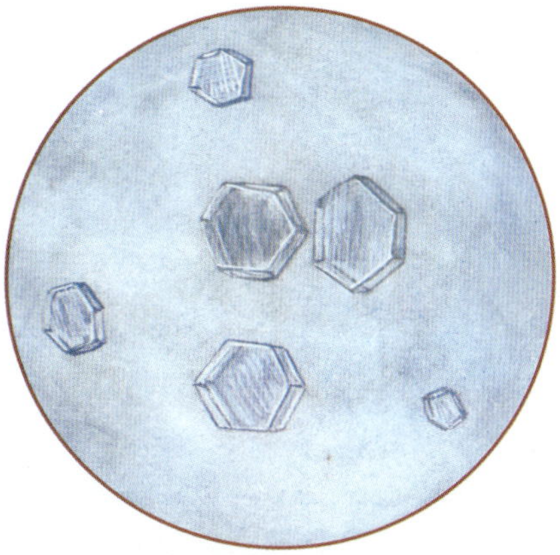

E, CYSTINE

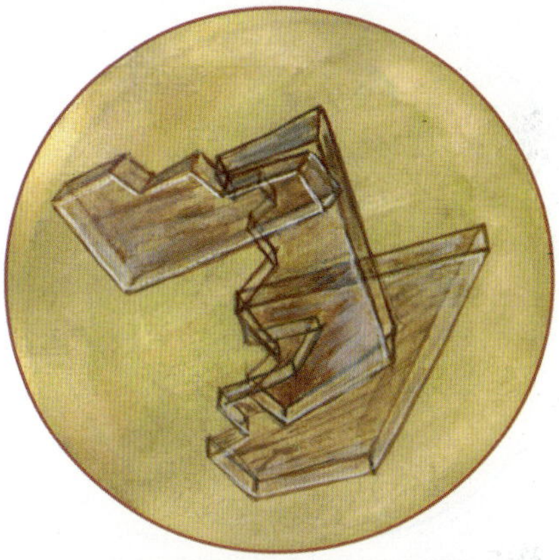

F, CHOLESTEROL

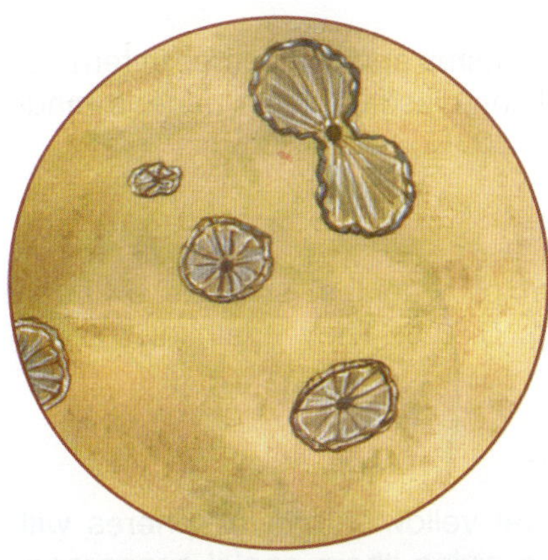

G, SULPHONAMIDE

FIGURE 6.4: Various types of crystals in acidic urine.

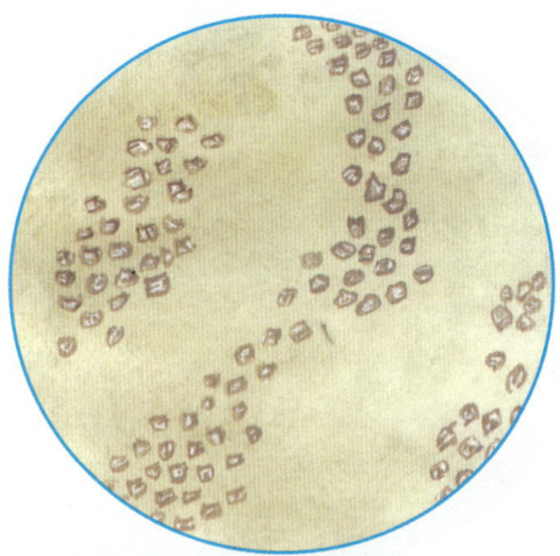

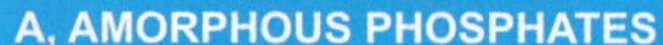

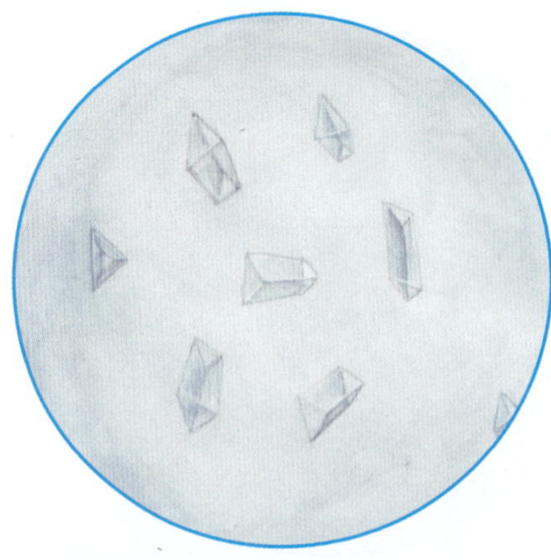

B, TRIPLE PHOSPHATES

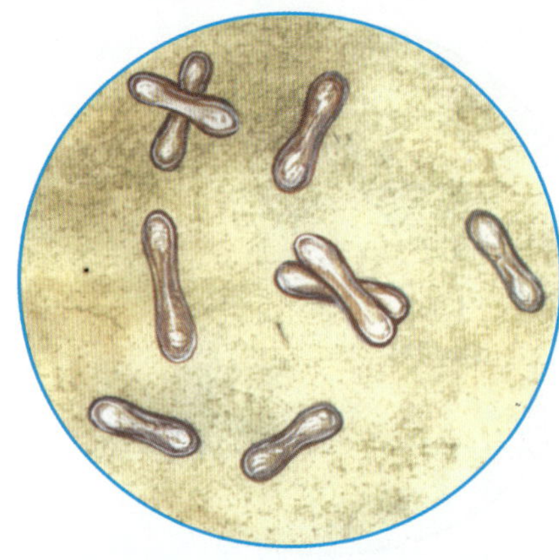

C, CALCIUM CARBONATE

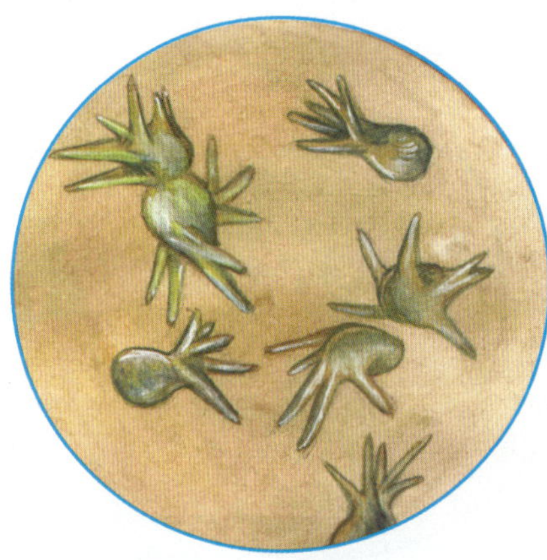

D, AMMONIUM BIURATES

FIGURE 6.5: Various types of crystals in alkaline urine.

vii) Sulphonamide

They appear as yellowish sheaves, rosettes, or rounded with radial striations (Fig. 6.4,G). They appear in urine after administration of sulphonamide drugs.

Crystals in Alkaline Urine

These are as under (Fig. 6.5):

i. Amorphous phosphate
ii. Triple phosphate
iii. Calcium carbonate
iv. Ammonium biurate

i) Amorphous Phosphate

They are seen as colourless granules in the form of clumps or irregular aggregates (Fig. 6.5,A). They dissolve when urine is made acidic.

ii) Triple Phosphate

They are in the form of prisms and sometimes in fern leaf pattern (Fig. 6.5,B). They dissolve when urine is made acidic.

iii) Calcium Carbonate

They are in the form of granules, spheres or rarely dumbbell-shaped (Fig. 5.5,C). They again dissolve in acidic urine.

iv) Ammonium Biurate

They are round or oval yellowish-brown spheres with thorns on their surface giving 'thorn apple' appearance (Fig. 6.5,D). They dissolve on heating the urine or by making it acidic.

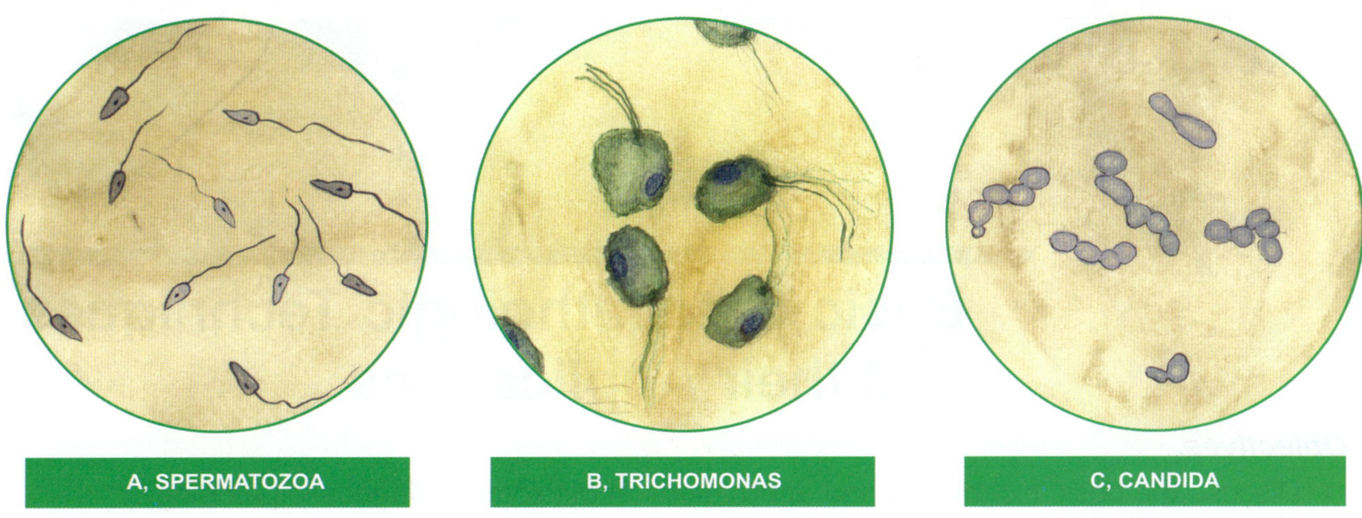

FIGURE 6.6: Miscellaneous structures in urine.

4. Miscellaneous Structures in Urine

These include the following (Fig. 6.6):

i. Spermatozoa
ii. Parasite
iii. Fungus
iv. Tumour cells

i) Spermatozoa

They can be seen in normal urine in males. They have a head and tail and can be motile (Fig. 6.6,A).

ii) Parasites

Urine may contain *Trichomonas vaginalis* which is more common in females (Fig. 6.6,B). Eggs of *Schistosoma hematobium* or *Entamoeba histolytica* can also be seen in urine.

iii) Fungus

Candida which are budding yeast cells can be seen in urine in patients with UTI or as contaminant (Fig. 6.6,C).

iv) Tumour Cells

Tumour cells having all the characteristics of malignancy may be seen singly or in groups in urine. These tumour cells could be from kidney, ureter, bladder or urethra. These cells are examined after staining of urine sediment.

D. AUTOMATION IN URINE ANALYSIS

In the recent times, automated urine analysis has been made possible by one of the following techniques:

Urine Strip Analysers

These are commercially available electronic urine strip readers. These strips may include various parameters of physical, chemical and microscopic constituents. After analysis, the results are obtained as print-out.

Flow Cytometry

Just as flow cytometry is used for blood and other body fluids, urine can be analysed by flow cytometry. In this method, DNA and membranes of formed elements are stained and pass as a laminar flow through a laser beam and the light scatter is measured by fluorescence impedance.

Exercise

7

Basic Cytopathologic Techniques and their Applications

Objectives

- Discuss the basic techniques and applications of cytology in diagnostic pathology.
- Illustrate a few common examples of exfoliative and fine needle aspiration cytology (FNAC).

Cytology is the study of body cells that are either exfoliated spontaneously from epithelial surfaces or are obtained from various body tissues and organs by different techniques. Currently, cytology has following branches:

A. Exfoliative cytology
B. Aspiration cytology
C. Imprint cytology

EXFOLIATIVE CYTOLOGY

This is the study of cells which are spontaneously shed off from epithelial surfaces into body cavities or fluid. The cells can also be obtained by scraping, brushing or wash of body surfaces. The principle of this technique is that in diseased states, rate of exfoliation of cells is increased.

Applications of Exfoliative Cytology

Exfoliative cytology is applied in diagnosing diseases of the following:

1. Female genital tract
2. Respiratory tract
3. Gastrointestinal tract
4. Urinary tract
5. Body fluids (pleural, peritoneal, pericardial, CSF and semen)
6. Buccal smears for sex chromatin

Female Genital Tract

Smears from female genital tract are known as 'Pap smears'. These smears are prepared by different methods depending upon the purpose for which they are intended:

i. *Cervical smear* It is obtained by Ayre's spatula (Fig. 7.1) from portio of the cervix by rotating the spatula through 360° to sample the entire cervix. The scraped material is placed on a clean glass

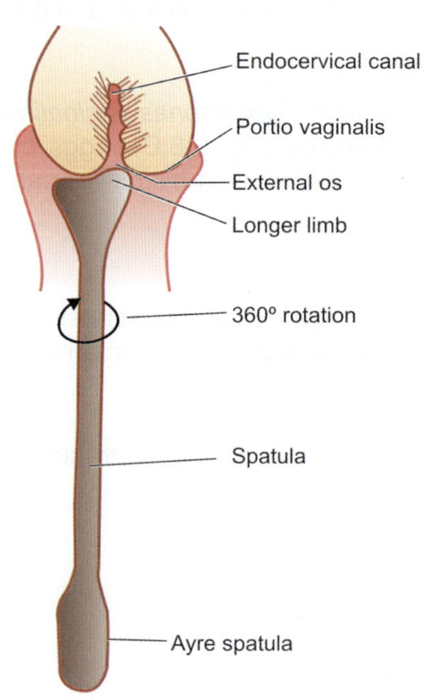

FIGURE 7.1: Method of obtaining cervical material for Fast smears.

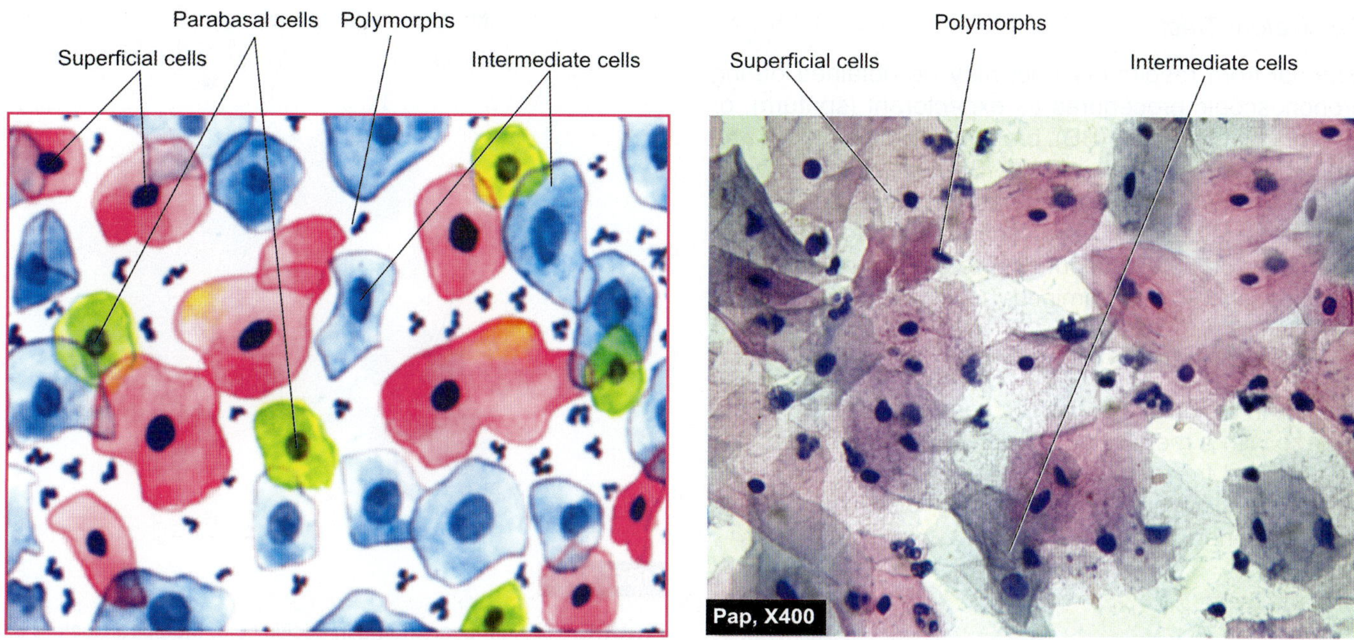

FIGURE 7.2: Pap smear, inflammatory. The field shows mainly superficial and some intermediate cells, and a few polymorphs.

slide and smear prepared. It is ideal for detection of cervical carcinoma.

ii. *Lateral vaginal smear (LVS)* is obtained by scraping upper third of lateral walls of the vagina and is ideal for cytohormonal assessment.

iii. *Vaginal pool smear* is obtained by aspirating material from posterior fornix of vagina and is done for detecting endometrial and ovarian carcinoma.

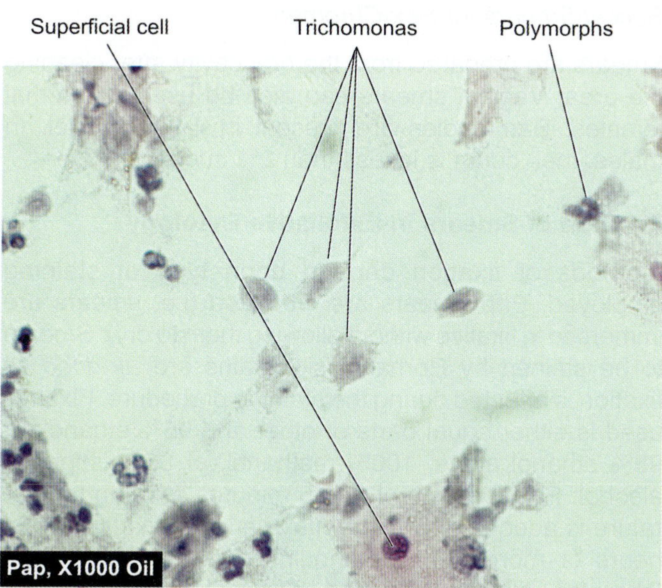

FIGURE 7.3: Pap smear showing *Trichomonas* vaginitis.

Salient microscopic features in Pap smear in inflammatory smear, trichomoniasis of the vagina and cervical cancer are shown in Figs 7.2 to 7.4.

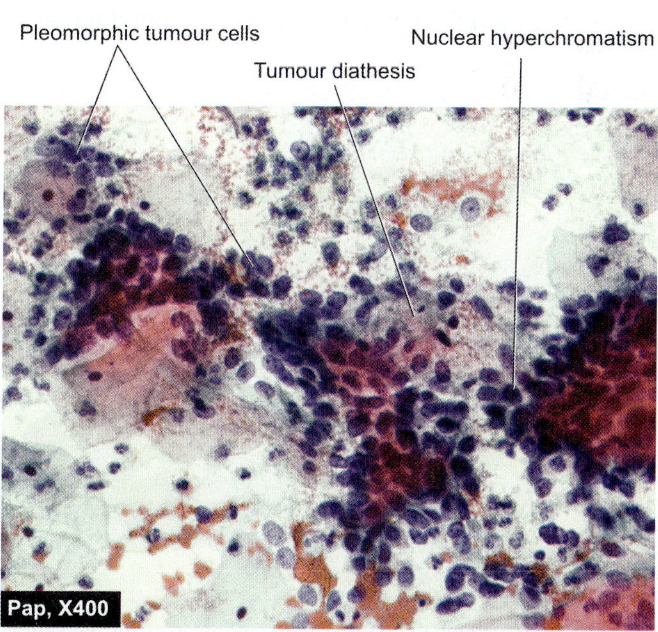

FIGURE 7.4: Pap smear in invasive carcinoma cervix. The field shows pleomorphic squamous cells in a sheet having coarse nuclear chromatin and some tumour diathesis in the background.

Respiratory Tract

Material from respiratory tract may be obtained during bronchoscopic procedures as expectorant (sputum), or by bronchial brushing (BB), bronchial washing (BW) and bronchioalveolar lavage (BAL). Sputum examination is advantageous as samples are easily obtained and cellular content is representative of entire respiratory tract. At least three samples of sputum, preferably early morning samples, should be examined.

Gastrointestinal Tract

Lesions in the oral cavity can be sampled by scraping the surface with a metallic or wooden spatula. Samples can be obtained from the oesophagus, stomach, small and large intestine either by brushing or lavage during fibreoptic endoscopy.

Urinary Tract

Samples from lesions in the urinary tract are either urinary sediment examined from voided urine/ catheterised urine or washings of the urinary bladder obtained at cystoscopy.

Body Fluids

Fluid from pleural, peritoneal or pericardial cavity is obtained by paracentesis. At least 50-100 ml of fluid is aspirated. The sample is examined fresh but if delay is anticipated then fluid should be anticoagulated either in EDTA 1 mg/ml or 3.8% sodium citrate 1 ml/10 ml. Fluid should be centrifuged and smears are prepared from the sediment. If amount of fluid is less (less than 1 ml), then it can be subjected to cytospin centrifuged smear preparation (Fig. 7.5).

Microscopic features of ascitic fluid in malignancy are shown in Fig. 7.6.

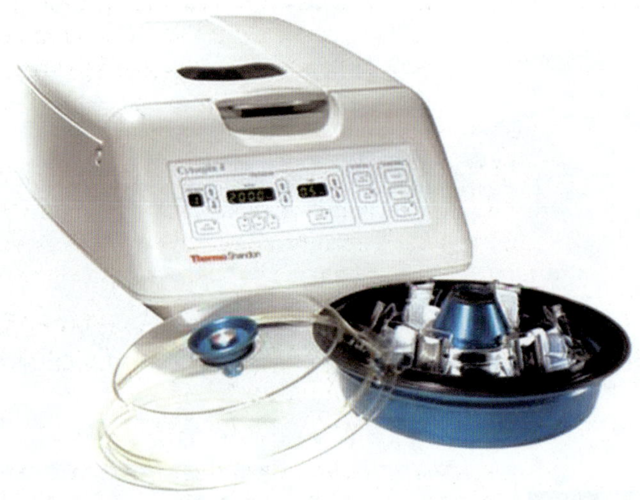

FIGURE 7.5: Cytospin used for making smears in cases with small volume of fluid (Photograph courtesy of Thermo Shandon, UK through Towa Optics India Pvt. Ltd., Delhi).

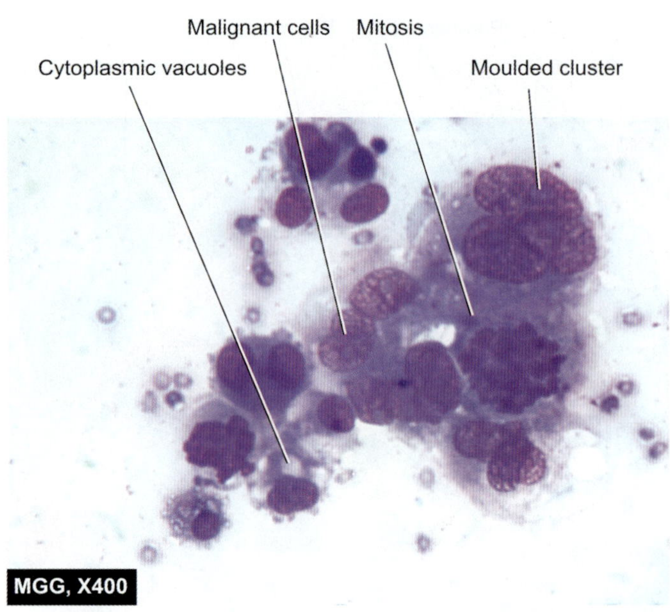

FIGURE 7.6: Adenocarcinoma in ascitic fluid. Moulded clusters of malignant cells seen with prominent nucleoli.

Buccal Smears for Sex Chromatin

Smears are prepared from the oral cavity after cleaning the area. Vaginal smears can also be used. In normal females, Barr bodies are present in 4-20% nuclei. In males, their count is in less than 2% nuclei.

Fixation of Smears in Exfoliative Cytology

Methods of fixation depend upon type of staining employed. Pap smears are *wet-fixed* (i.e. smears are immersed in fixative without allowing them to dry). Smears to be stained by Romanowsky stains are *air-dried* as fixation is affected during the staining procedure. Fixative used is either equal parts of ether and 95% ethanol, or 95% ethanol alone, 100% methanol, or 85% isopropyl alcohol. Fixation time of 10-15 minutes at room temperature is adequate. Smears may be left in fixative for 24 hours or more. Smears should be transported to the laboratory in fixative solution in coplin jars.

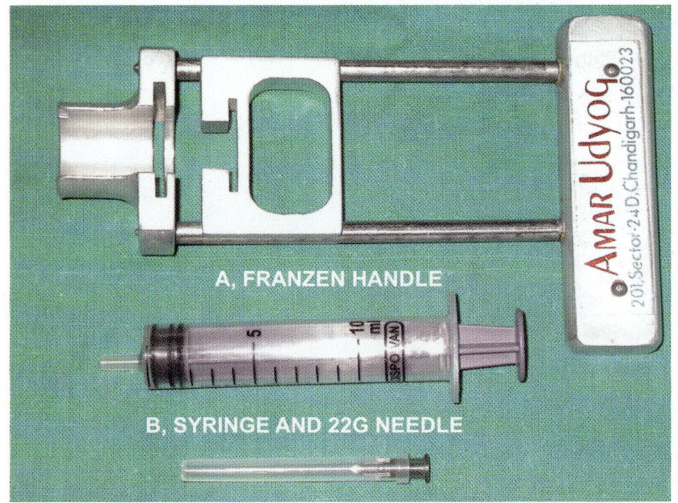

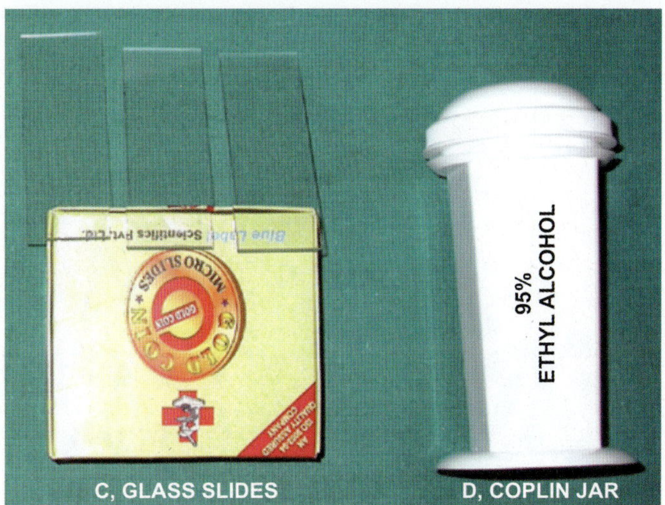

FIGURE 7.7: Equipment required for transcutaneous FNAC.

Staining of Smears in Exfoliative Cytology

Three staining procedures are commonly employed: Papanicolaou and H and E stains are used for *wet-fixed smears* while Romanowsky stains are used for *air-dried smears*.

Papanicolaou Stain

This is the best stain for routine cytodiagnostic studies. In this, haematoxylin gives nuclear stain while OG-6 and EA-50 are two cytoplasmic counterstains.

H and E Stain

This is the same as that used for histological sections. In this, haematoxylin is nuclear stain and eosin is cytoplasmic counterstain.

Romanowsky Stain

Leishman's stain, Giemsa and May-Grünwald-Giemsa (MGG) are used; the last one is most commonly used.

ASPIRATION CYTOLOGY

In this study, samples are obtained from diseased tissue by fine needle aspiration (FNA).

Applications of FNA

FNA is applied for diagnosis of palpable as well as non-palpable lesions.

I. Palpable Mass Lesions in:

1. Lymph nodes
2. Breast
3. Thyroid
4. Salivary glands
5. Soft tissue masses
6. Bones

II. Non-Palpable Mass Lesions in:

1. Abdominal cavity
2. Thoracic cavity
3. Retroperitoneum

Procedure for FNA

Materials For performing FNA, a Franzen's handle, syringe with needles, clean glass slides and suitable fixative are required (Fig. 7.7).

A few prototype examples of applications of FNA are shown in Figs 7.8 to 7.10. These are: tuberculous lymphadenitis, fibroadenoma breast and breast cancer.

Radiological Imaging Aids for FNA

Non-palpable lesions require some form of localisation by radiological aids for FNA to be carried out. Plain X-ray is usually adequate for lesions in bones and chest. Ultrasonography (USG) allows direct visualisation of needle in intra-abdominal and soft tissue masses. CT scan can be used for lesions in chest and abdomen.

Advantages of FNA over Surgical Biopsy

i. Outdoor procedure
ii. No anaesthesia required
iii. Results obtained within hours
iv. Procedure can be repeated
v. Low cost procedure

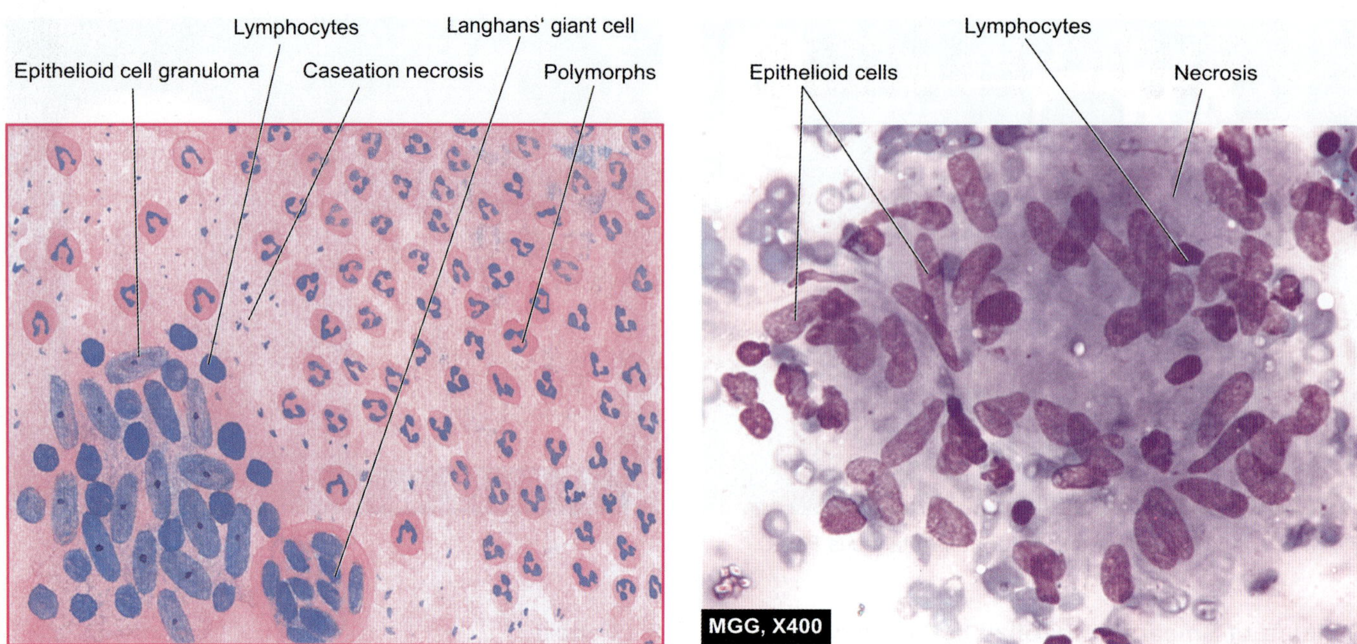

FIGURE 7.8: FNA smear from tuberculous lymphadenitis. There are epithelioid cell clusters and necrotic debris in the background.

IMPRINT CYTOLOGY

In imprint cytology, touch preparations from cut surfaces of fresh unfixed surgically excised tissue are prepared on clean glass slides. These are fixed, stained and examined immediately. It is considered complementary to frozen section.

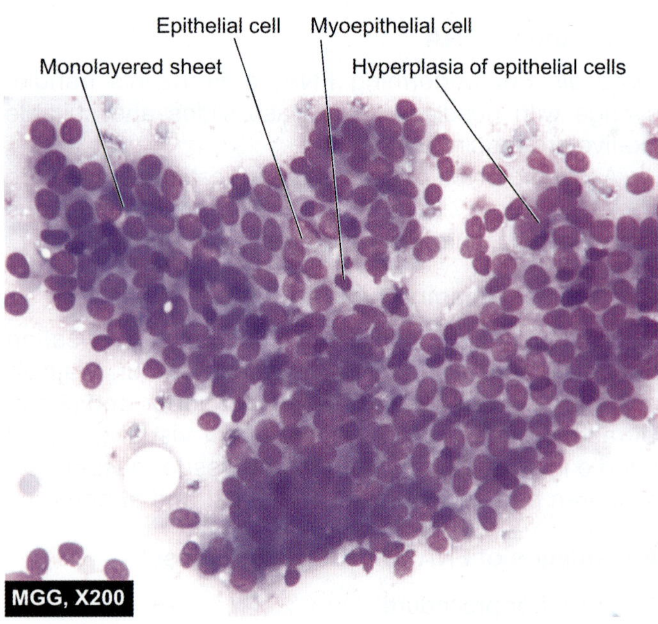

FIGURE 7.9: FNA breast from fibroadenoma breast. The field shows monolayered sheet of monomorphic cells and some fibromyxoid stromal fragment.

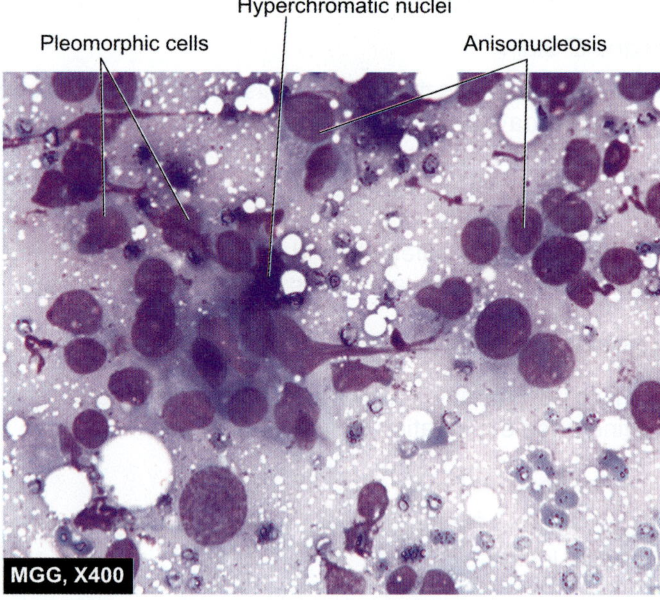

FIGURE 7.10: FNA breast, duct carcinoma. Scattered pleomorphic malignant cells with hyperchromatic nuclei.

Section Three

HAEMATOLOGY

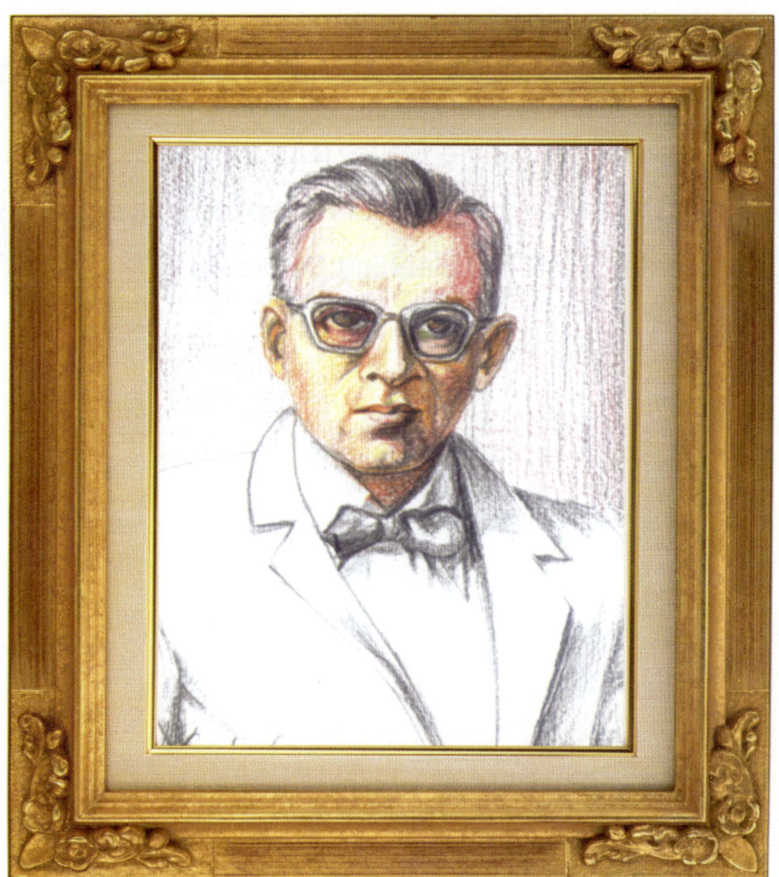

MM WINTROBE (1901–1986)

American Physician, who devised Wintrobe haematocrit tube for estimation of PCV and ESR and thus enabled measuring red cell indices. Wintrobe was a pupil of William Loyd, a pioneering teacher and eminent author of last century, and regarded him as a very stimulating teacher.

Section Contents

Exercise

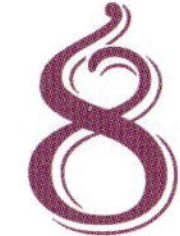

Haemoglobin Estimation—Various Methods

Objectives

- ⇨ Discuss the various methods for estimation of haemoglobin.
- ⇨ Briefly comment on the concept of quality control in haemoglobin estimation.

Haemoglobin (Hb) is the main component of red blood cells and is a conjugated protein. A molecule of Hb contains two pairs of polypeptide chains α_2 β_2 and four haem groups each having an atom of ferrous iron. The oxygen-carrying capacity of Hb when fully saturated is 1.34 ml/g. Approximately 34% of the RBCs by weight is Hb. Iron content of Hb is 0.347 gm/100 g. The main function of Hb is to transport oxygen from lungs to the tissues. There are various forms of Hb as under :

i. Oxyhaemoglobin (HbO_2)
ii. Carboxy haemoglobin (HbCO)
iii. Sulfhaemoglobin (SHb)
iv. Methaemoglobin (Hi)

The measurement of concentration of Hb in the blood is known as haemoglobinometry.

Types of blood samples used for Hb estimation are as under:

i. *Capillary blood* from finger prick.
ii. *Intravenous sample*—It should be well anticoagulated, preferably in EDTA. Liquid anticoagulants should not be used at all as these dilute and decrease Hb concentration.

METHODS FOR ESTIMATION OF HAEMOGLOBIN

Various methods used for estimation of Hb are divided into 4 groups as under:

I. Colorimetric method: Colorimetric method is based on colorimetric measurement of the intensity of colour developed on addition of some substance to the blood. Colorimetric methods include the following:

1. Cyanmethaemoglobin method
2. Oxyhaemoglobin method
3. Electronic counter method
4. Direct reading electronic haemoglobinometer
5. Sahli's method

II. Measurement of O_2 carrying capacity of Hb: Measurement of O_2 carrying capacity of Hb cannot be used for mass screening but is used in referral or research laboratories only.

III. Measurement of iron content of Hb: Measurement of iron content of Hb is used only for research purpose.

IV. Specific gravity method: It is a very rapid method and is useful for screening blood donors for anaemia in blood donation programme. Normal specific gravity of blood ranges from 1.048-1.066.

Some of the commonly used methods are discussed below.

Cyanmet Hb Method

This is the best method for Hb estimation and it has been recommended by International Committee for Standardisation in Haematology (ICSH).

Principle Blood is diluted in a solution called Drabkin's fluid containing potassium ferricyanide and potassium cyanide (KCN). The oxy, carboxy and metHb are all converted into cyanmet Hb (HiCN) and there is development of pink colour. The intensity of pink colour can be measured in a spectrophotometer or photoelectric colorimeter at 540 nm and this is compared with that of a standard cyanmethaemoglobin solution.

Reagents Drabkin's fluid can be prepared as under:

Potassium ferricyanide	:	0.2 g
Potassium cyanide	:	0.05 g
Dihydrogen potassium phosphate	:	0.14 g
Distilled water	:	1000 ml

Drabkin's fluid should be clear and pale yellow having a pH of 7.0-7.4.

Procedure

- Add 20 μl (0.02 ml) of blood to 5 ml of Drabkin's solution in a test tube (1:251 dilution).
- Mix well and allow it to stand for 3-5 minutes.
- Take reading of test and standard in a spectrophotometer or photoelectric colorimeter at 540 nm (Fig. 8.1).

Calculations

Hb concentration in test (g%) =

$$\frac{\text{Absorbance of test}}{\text{Absorbance of standard}} \times \frac{\text{Hb concentration of standard (mg/dl)} \times 251}{100 \text{ mg/g}}$$

Where 251 is the dilution factor.

Advantages

i. There is no chance of visual error.
ii. All forms of Hb except sulfhaemoglobin can be measured.
iii. The standard is very stable.

Disadvantages

i. We cannot take the reading immediately.
ii. If blood is turbid due to plasma proteins, hyperlipidaemia or leukaemias, the absorbance is more and hence incorrect results may be obtained.
iii. Results are affected due to hyperbilirubinaemia.

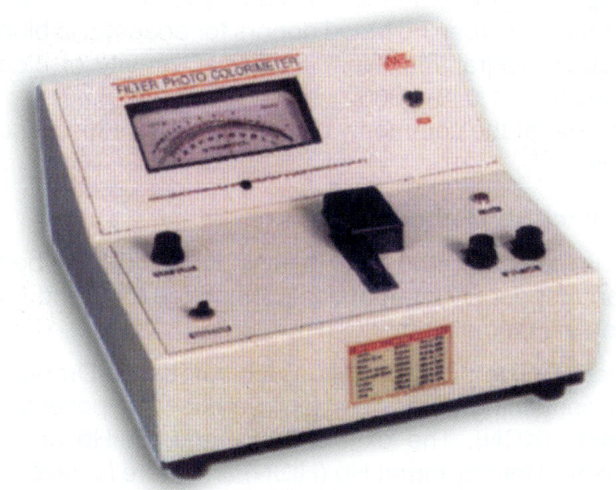

FIGURE 8.1: Photoelectric colorimeter used for taking reading of haemoglobin in cyanmet Hb method and oxyhaemoglobin method. (Photograph courtesy of Max Electronics India, Chandigarh).

Oxyhaemoglobin Method

This is a simple and quick method and results are not affected by hyperbilirubinaemia.

Principle Blood is diluted in a solution of ammonia. There is development of reddish pink-colour which is measured in a spectrophotometer or photoelectric colorimeter at 625 nm and compared with that of a standard oxyHb solution.

Procedure

- Add 20 μl (0.02 ml) of blood to 4 ml of 0.4 ml/l ammonia solution in a test tube.
- Use a tight fitting stopper and mix by inverting the tube several times.
- Take reading of test and standard in a spectrophotometer or photoelectric colorimeter with a yellow or green filter (625 nm).

Calculations As for cyanmet method.

Advantages

i. The method is simple and quick.
ii. Result is not affected by rise of plasma bilirubin.
iii. Most forms of haemoglobins (i.e. HbO, Hi, and HbCO) are measured in this method.

Disadvantages

i. It does not measure sulfhaemoglobin.
ii. The standard is not stable.
iii. Increased absorbance may be caused by turbidity due to hyperlipidaemia, leucocytosis (> 30×10^9/L) and abnormal plasma proteins.

Electronic Counter Method

This is a multi-parameter determining electronic equipment.

Principle The method is based on electrical impedance principle. The blood is diluted with isoton and lysate which lyses the RBCs converting Hb into cyanmethaemaglobin and its concentration is measured in the spectrophotometer at 540 nm. In some instruments, cyanmethaemoglobin method is replaced with another method employing a non-toxic chemical, sodium lauryl sulphate.

Disadvantage

i. High white cell count (> 30,000/μl) produces false elevation of Hb.

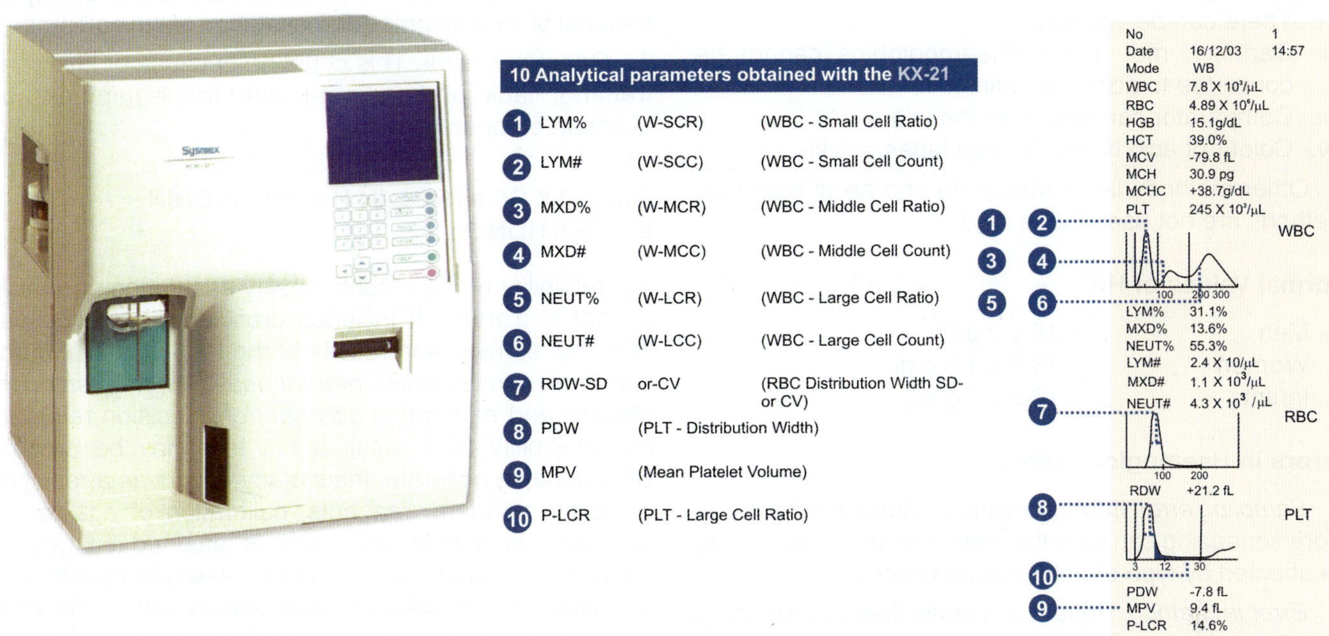

FIGURE 8.2: Electronic particle counter (Haematology Analyser) Model K X –21 (Photograph courtesy of Sysmex Corporation, Japan through Transasia Biomedicals Ltd., Mumbai).

Direct Reading Electronic Haemoglobinometers

These have inbuilt filters. Reading of Hb in g/dl is visualised on the screen which may have light emitting diode (LED) display or analog meter. These equipments work on the principle of cyanmetHb, oxyHb method or colour comparators in which colour of blood is compared without conversion to a derivative, against a range of colours which represent haemoglobin concentration (Fig. 8.2).

Disadvantage

i. Calibration of the instrument can be faulty.

Sahli's Method

Principle Hb is converted into acid haematin with the action of dilute hydrochloric acid (N/10 HCl). The acid haematin is brown in colour and its intensity is matched with a standard brown glass comparator in a visual colorimeter called Sahli's colorimeter.

Procedure

- Fill Sahli's Hb tube upto mark 2 with N/10 HCl.
- Deliver 20 µl (0.02 ml) of blood from a Hb pipette into it.
- Stir with a stirrer and wait for 10 minutes.
- Add distilled water drop by drop and stir till colour matches with the comparator.
- Take the reading at upper meniscus (Fig. 8.3).

Advantages

i. Simple bedside test.
ii. Reagents and apparatus are cheap.

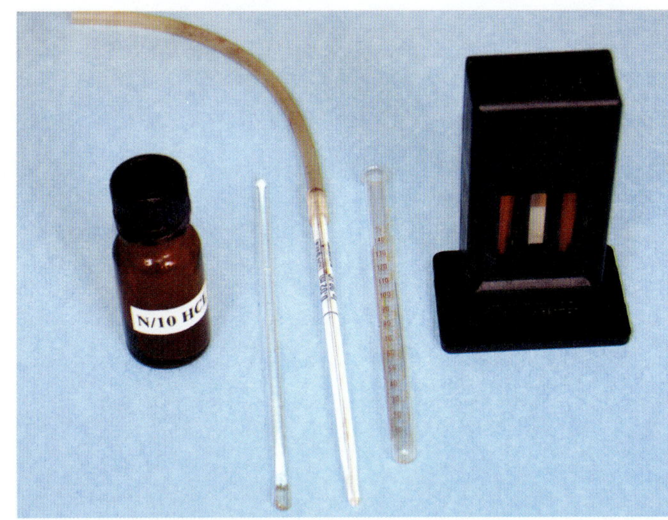

FIGURE 8.3: Apparatus used for Sahli's haemoglobinometry.

Disadvantages

i. There can be visual error.
ii. Carboxy, met and sulfhaemoglobins cannot be converted to acid haematin.
iii. Comparator can fade over the years.
iv. Colour of acid haematin also fades quickly.

Other methods like carboxy Hb and alkali haematin methods are not used these days.

Normal Values of Hb

Men	:	15 ± 2 g/dl
Women	:	13.5 ± 1.5 g/dl
Infants	:	16.5 ± 3 g/dl

Errors in Haemoglobinometry

1. *Sampling error:* Improper venipuncture technique e.g. more squeezing can alter the results, or the reading may be affected by type of anticoagulant used.

2. *Error in method:* Results are better with cyanmet and oxy Hb method. In Sahli's method, chances of error are more.

3. *Error in equipment:* These could be due to quality of material of the equipment or calibration of the equipment.

4. *Operator's error:* This could be because of improper training, lack of familiarity with the equipment or overworked operator.

QUALITY CONTROL IN HAEMOGLOBIN ESTIMATION

For reliability of the results, quality assurance or quality control is a must. It includes proficiency in collection, labelling, storage and results of the test. Quality control has three components: *internal quality control, standardisation* and *external quality control.* Precision refers to reproducibility of a result but a test may be precise without being accurate. Inaccuracy occurs as a result of improper standard, reagents, calibration of equipment and poor technique. Accuracy is attained by use of reference material which has been assayed by different methods and in different laboratories. The reference materials are commercially available with known values of results, or can be prepared in the laboratory.

Exercise

9

Counting of Blood Cells

Objectives

- ⇨ Discuss the principle, techniques and interpretation of WBC, RBC and platelet counts.
- ⇨ Comment on their normal values and conditions producing abnormal counts of these blood cells.

WBC COUNT

This is determination of number of white blood cells per µl of blood.

Methods

There are two methods:

1. Visual haemacytometer method
2. Electronic method

Visual Haemacytometer Method

Principle This is counting of WBCs in a calibrated chamber by diluting of blood to 1:20 dilution with diluent which causes lysis of RBCs and staining of WBCs.

Diluting fluid Turk's fluid is used which has the following composition :

Glacial acetic acid	:	3.0 ml
1% Aqueous gentian violet	:	2.0 ml
Distilled water	:	195 ml

Procedure

- ◆ Suck anticoagulated blood or blood from finger prick upto mark 0.5 in WBC pipette (Fig. 9.1,A).
- ◆ Wipe tip and outside of the pipette.
- ◆ Draw diluting fluid upto mark 11 in the WBC pipette.
- ◆ Mix well by rotating the pipette for 2-3 minutes.
- ◆ Charge the Neubauer's chamber after discarding 1-2 drops of the mixture from the WBC pipette.
- ◆ Allow the cells to settle down for 2 minutes.
- ◆ Count the WBCs under low power (10x) in 4 large corner squares (Fig. 9.2). Count the cells lying on left and lower lines while ignoring those on its right and upper lines.

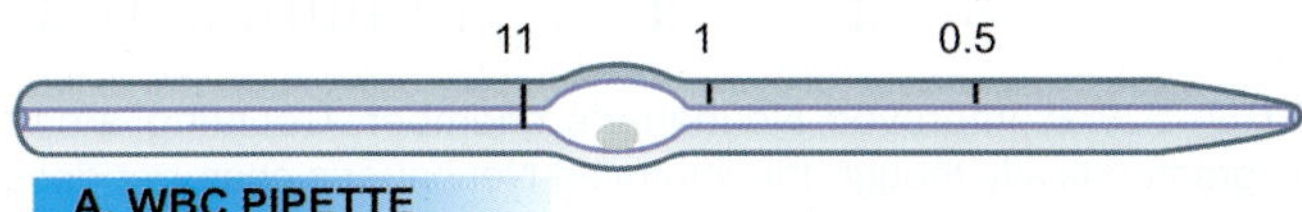

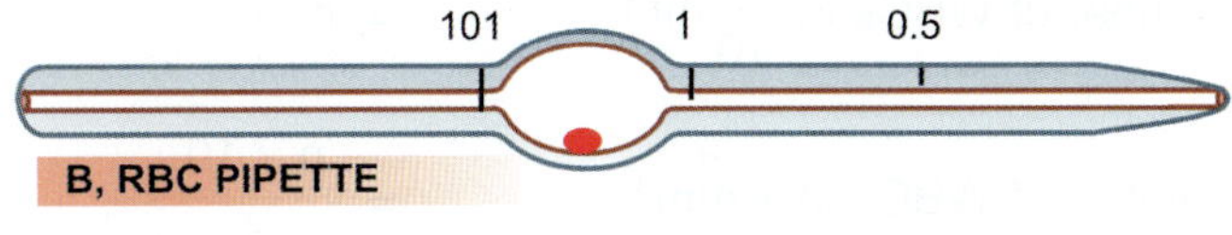

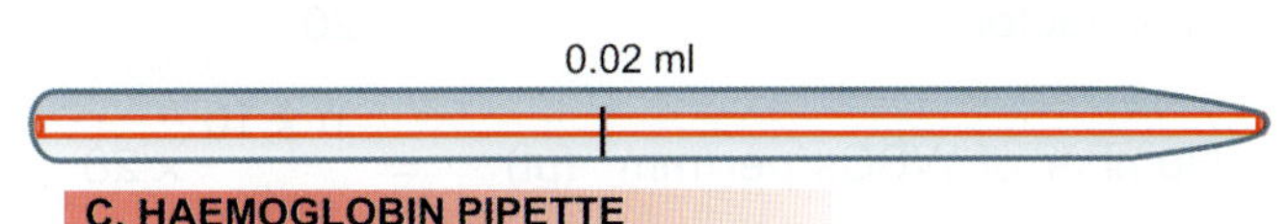

FIGURE 9.1: Pipettes for WBC (A) and RBC counting (B) contrasted with haemoglobin pipette (C).

*Calculations**

Volume of area in which WBCs counted in 4 corner squares $= [(1 \times 1 \times 0.1) \times 4]\ mm^3$

$$= \frac{4}{10} mm^3$$

*For calculation of count of WBCs, RBCs and platelets using Neubauer's chamber, please remember the dimensions of corner squares of the chamber as 1 mm each side and depth 0.1 mm. Volume = Length × Breadth × Depth

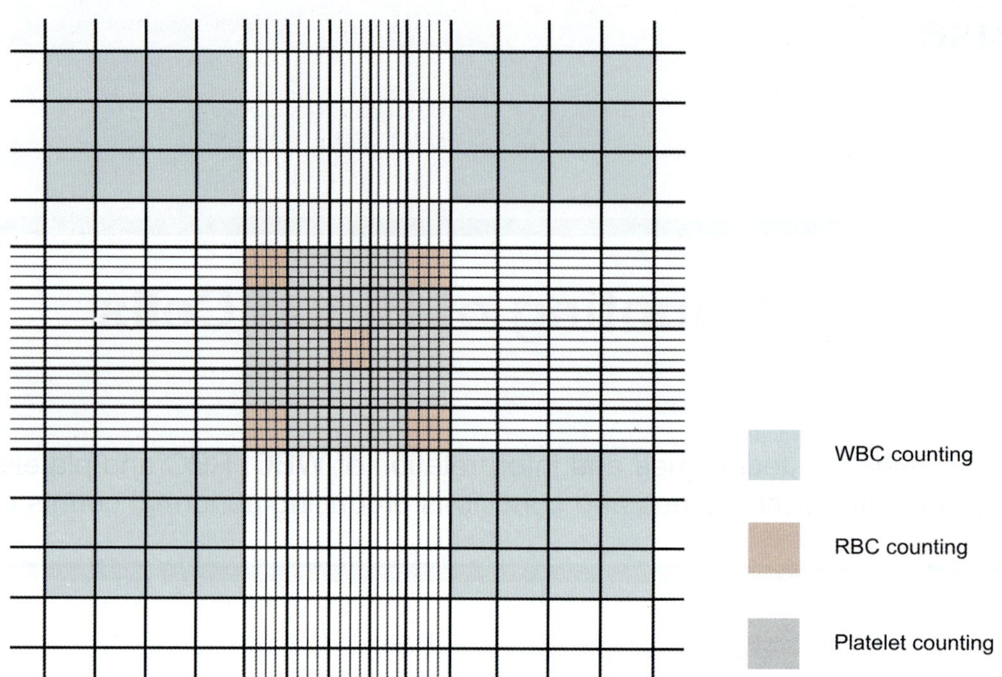

FIGURE 9.2: Improved Neubauer's chamber. Counting areas for WBCs, RBCs and platelets are depicted by different colours diagrammatically though the improved Neubauer's chamber does not have any such colours.

Number of WBCs in $\frac{4}{10}$ mm^3 $= n$

Number of WBCs in 1 mm^3 $= \frac{n \times 10}{4}$

Dilution factor $= 20$

$\therefore$ Number of WBCs per mm^3 (µl) $= \frac{n \times 10}{4} \times 20$

$= n \times 50$

where n is the total number of WBCs counted in 4 corner squares.

Precautions

i. The work bench must be free of vibrations and chamber should not be exposed to heat.
ii. The cover glass should be of special thickness and should have perfectly flat surface.
iii. The chamber area should be completely filled leaving no air bubbles or debris in the chamber area.
iv. The fluid should not overflow to the moat.

Electronic Method

Electronic counter is based on the principle of aperture impedance method, or light scattering technology, or both. In this, particles passing through a chamber in single file scatter the light and convert by a detector into pulses proportionate to the size of the cells, which are then counted electronically. A lysate is used to lyse red cells so as to count WBCs.

Advantages

i. Easy and rapid method.
ii. Time saving method.
iii. Very large number of cells are counted rapidly.
iv. There is high level of precision.

Disadvantages

i. Costly equipment.
ii. Calibration error.
iii. Nucleated RBCs are counted as leucocytes.
iv. Platelet clumps counted as leucocytes.

Normal Range for WBC Count

Adults : 4,000–11,000/µl
Infants at birth : 10,000–26,000/µl
Children under 1 year : 6,000–18,000/µl

Causes of Abnormal Leucocyte Count

Increased leucocyte count – Leucocytosis
Decreased leucocyte count – Leucopenia

The conditions causing *leucocytosis* and *leucopenia* are given in Exercise 11.

RBC COUNT

This is defined as determination of the number of RBCs per µl of blood.

Methods for RBC Counts

1. Visual haemacytometer method
2. Electronic method

Visual Haemacytometer Method

Principle This is counting of RBCs in a calibrated chamber by dilution of blood to 1 in 200 dilution with a diluent which is isotonic to blood. The diluent used prevents clotting, clumping and rouleaux formation and does not destroy WBCs.

Diluting fluids
Two types of diluting fluids are used for RBC counting: Hayem's fluid and Dacie's fluid.

Composition of Hayem's fluid

Mercuric chloride	:	0.25 g
Sodium chloride	:	0.5 g
Sodium sulphate	:	2.5 g
Distilled water	:	100 ml

Composition of Dacie's fluid

40% Formaldehyde	:	5 ml
3% Trisodium citrate	:	495 ml

Procedure
- Draw anticoagulated blood or blood from finger prick upto mark 0.5 in RBC pipette (Fig. 9.1,B).
- Wipe tip and outside of the pipette.
- Draw diluting fluid upto mark 101 in the RBC pipette.
- Mix well by rotating the pipette for 2-3 minutes.
- Charge the Neubauer's chamber after discarding 1-2 drops of mixture from the RBC pipette.
- Allow the cells to settle down for 2 minutes.
- Count RBCs under high power 40X in 80 tiny squares (5 × 16 tiny squares) in the centre of the chamber as shown in Fig. 9.2.

Calculations
Volume of area in which RBCs counted in 5 squares

$$= \left[\left(\frac{1}{5}\times\frac{1}{5}\times 0.1\right)\times 5\right] mm^3$$

$$= \frac{1}{50} mm^3$$

$\therefore$ Number of RBCs in volume $\frac{1}{50} mm^3 = n$

Number of RBCs in 1 mm^3	= n x 50
Dilution factor	= 200
$\therefore$ RBC count per mm^3 (µl)	= n x 50 x 200
	= n x 10,000

Where n is the number of RBCs counted in 5 small squares.

Electronic Method

Principle Principle of electronic method for counting RBCs is the same as for WBCs. But unlike WBC counting, no lysate is used; instead anticoagulated blood is diluted with particle-free diluting fluid such as physiological saline or phosphate buffer saline.

Advantages
i. Easy and rapid method.
ii. Many thousands of cells are counted compared to fewer cells counted in manual method.

Disadvantages
i. Costly equipment.
ii. Calibration error.
iii. Altered composition of diluent causes erroneous results.
iv. Giant platelets are counted as RBCs.
v. High WBC count alters results.

Normal Range for RBC Count

Males	:	5.0–6.0 million/µl (5.5 $\pm$ 0.5 million/µl)
Females	:	4.5–5.5 million/µl (5 $\pm$ 0.5 million/µl)
Children	:	4.0–5.0 million/µl (4.5 $\pm$ 0.5 million/µl)

Cause of Decreased RBC Count

i. Anaemia

Cause of Increased RBC Count

i. Polycythemia

PLATELET COUNT

Platelets are thin discs 2-4 µm in diameter. They function in haemostasis, in maintaining vascular integrity and in the process of blood coagulation. Their life span is 7-10 days.

Methods for Counting Platelets

1. Visual method
2. Electronic method

Visual Method

Type of blood used Use only venous blood as the blood obtained from finger prick causes clumping of platelets.
Diluting fluid 1% ammonium oxalate is prepared as under:

Ammonium oxalate	:	1g
Distilled water	:	100 ml

Filter it and keep in a refrigerator at 4°C.

Procedure

- Using an RBC pipette, prepare a 1:200 dilution as for RBC method (Fig. 9. i,B).
- Mix for 2 minutes, charge the Neubauer's counting chamber.
- Place the charged Neubauer's chamber into a petri dish having a moist filter paper at bottom for allowing the platelets to settle down.
- Count the platelets as for red cell count using 40x objective with reduced condenser aperture.
- If platelet count is low, a WBC pipette can be used for charging the Neubauer's chamber.

Calculations

Volume of area in which platelets counted in 5 squares

$$= \left[\left(\frac{1}{5}\times\frac{1}{5}\times 0.1\right)\times 5\right] mm^3$$

$$= \frac{1}{50} mm^3$$

$$\therefore \text{Number of platelets in volume } \frac{1}{50} mm^3 = n$$

Number of platelets in 1 mm^3 = n x 50
Dilution factor = 200
$\therefore$ Platelet count per mm^3 (µl) = n x 50 x 200
= n x 10,000

A phase contrast microscope can be used for platelet counting which gives better results.

Rough Visual Method for Platelet Counting

Prepare a thin peripheral blood film, stain it with any of the Romanowsky stain. Dry it and examine under high power. If you find one clump of platelet per high power field, then number of platelets is adequate; roughly each platelet under high power represents count of 25,000 platelets per mm^3.

Electronic Method

Platelets can be counted by electronic particle counter method which implies electrical impedance principle as for counting RBCs.

Disadvantages

i. Equipment is costly.
ii. Calibration error.
iii. Debris counted as platelets.
iv. Heinz bodies and Howell-Jolly bodies can be counted as platelets.

Normal Platelet Count

1,50,000-400,000/µl

Conditions causing abnormal platelet counts

Decreased count is termed thrombocytopenia
Increased count is termed thrombocytosis.

Conditions causing Thrombocytopenia

1. *Impaired platelet production:*
   i. Aplastic anaemia
   ii. Acute leukaemias
   iii. Myelofibrosis
   iv. Marrow infiltration by malignancy
   v. Drugs (e.g. chloramphenicol, thiazides, anticancer drugs)
   vi. Chronic alcoholism
2. *Accelerated platelet destruction:*
   i. ITP
   ii. SLE
   iii. AIDS
   iv. CLL
   v. DIC
   vi. Giant haemangioma
   vii. Drug-induced (e.g. sulfonamides, quinine, gold)
   viii. Microangiopathic haemolytic anaemia
   ix. Splenomegaly
   x. Massive transfusion of blood

Conditions Causing Thrombocytosis

i. Essential thrombocytosis
ii. Chronic infection
iii. Haemorrhage
iv. Post-operative state
v. Malignancy
vi. Post-splenectomy.

Exercise

10

Preparation and Staining of Peripheral Blood Film

Objectives

- ⇨ Discuss the technique and significance of thin and thick blood film.
- ⇨ Briefly comment on the various stains used for staining blood films.

The peripheral blood film (PBF) is of two types:
1. Thin blood film
2. Thick blood film

THIN BLOOD FILM

Thin PBF can be prepared from anticoagulated blood obtained by venepuncture or from free flowing finger prick blood by any of the following three techniques:
1. Slide method
2. Cover glass method
3. Spin method

Slide Method

Procedure

- Place a drop of blood in the centre of a clean glass slide 1 to 2 cm from one end.
- Place another slide (spreader) with smooth edge at an angle of 30-45° near the drop of blood.
- Move the spreader backward so that it makes contact with drop of blood.
- Then move the spreader forward rapidly over the slide.
- A thin peripheral blood film is thus prepared (Fig. 10.1).
- Dry it and stain it.

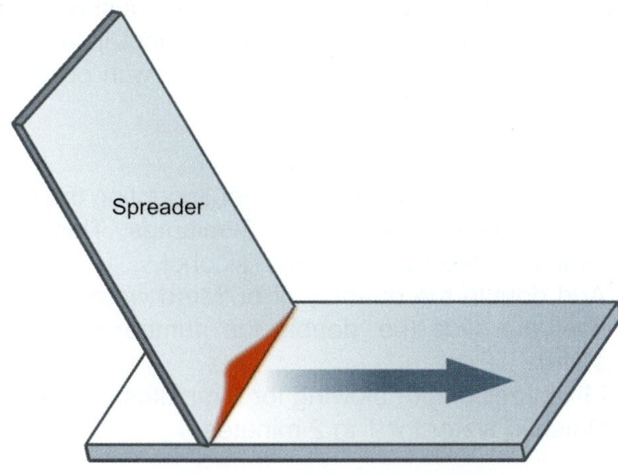

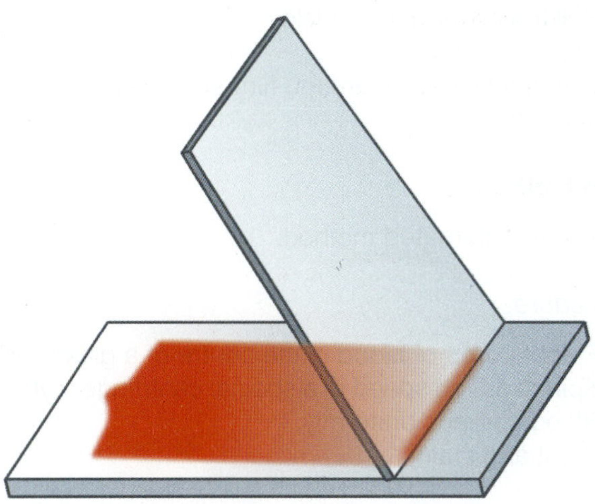

FIGURE 10.1: Method of making thin PBF by slide method.

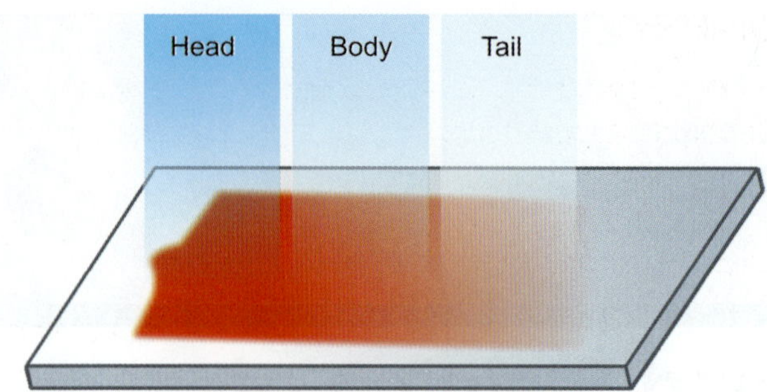

FIGURE 10.2: Parts of a thin blood film.

Qualities of a Good Blood Film

i. It should not cover the entire surface of slide.
ii. It should have smooth and even appearance.
iii. It should be free from waves and holes.
iv. It should not have irregular tail.

Parts of a Thin Blood Film

A PBF consists of 3 parts (Fig. 10.2):

1. *Head* i.e. the portion of blood film near the drop of blood.
2. *Body* i.e. the main part of the blood film.
3. *Tail* i.e. the tapering end of the blood film.

Cover Glass Method

Procedure

- Take a No.1 (22 mm square) clean cover glass.
- Touch it on to the drop of a blood.
- Place it on another similar cover glass in crosswise direction with side containing drop of blood facing down.
- Pull the cover glass quickly.
- Dry it and stain it.
- Mount it with a mountant, film side down on a clean glass slide.

Spin Method

This is an automated method.

Procedure

- Place a drop of blood in the centre of a glass slide.
- Spin at a high speed in a special centrifuge, cytospin.
- Blood spreads uniformly.
- Dry it and stain it.

THICK BLOOD FILM

This is prepared for detecting blood parasites such as malaria and microfilaria.

Procedure

- Place a large drop of blood in the centre of a clean glass slide.
- Spread it in a circular area of 1.5 cm with the help of a stick or end of another glass slide.
- Dry it and you should be able to just see the printed matter through the smear, when kept on printed paper.

STAINS FOR BLOOD FILM

Romanowsky stains are universally employed for staining of blood films. All Romanowsky combinations have two essential ingredients i.e. methylene blue and eosin or azure. Methylene blue is the basic dye and has affinity for acidic component of the cell (i.e. nucleus) and eosin/azure is the acidic dye and has affinity for basic component of cell (i.e. cytoplasm).

Most Romanowsky stains are prepared in methyl alcohol so that they combine fixation and staining.

Various stains included under Romanowsky stain are as under:

i. Leishman stain
ii. Giemsa stain
iii. Wright stain
iv. Field stain
v. Jenner stain
vi. JSB stain

Staining of Thin Blood Film

Leishman Stain

Preparation Dissolve 0.2 g of powdered Leishman's dye in 100 ml of acetone-free methyl alcohol in a conical flask. Warm it to 50°C for half an hour with occasional shaking. Cool it and filter it.

Procedure for staining

- Pour Leishman's stain dropwise (counting the drops) on the slide and wait for 2 minutes. This allows fixation of the PBF in methyl alcohol.
- Add double the quantity of buffered water dropwise over the slide (i.e. double the number of drops of stain).
- Mix by rocking or blowing for 8 minutes.
- Wash in water for 1 to 2 minutes.

- Dry in air and examine under oil immersion lens of the microscope.

Giemsa Stain

Preparation Stock solution of Giemsa stain is prepared by mixing 0.15 g of Giemsa powder in 12.5 ml of glycerine and 12.5 ml of methyl alcohol. Before use dissolve one volume of stock solution in nine volumes of buffered water (dilution 1:9).

Procedure

- Pour diluted stain over slide.
- Wait for 15-60 minutes.
- Wash in water.
- Dry it and examine under oil immersion lens of the microscope.

Staining of Thick Smear

It can be stained with any of the Romanowsky stains listed above except that before staining, the smear is dehaemoglobinised by putting it in distilled water for 10 minutes.

Autostainers

Currently, automatic staining machines are available which enable a large batch of slides to be stained with a uniform quality.

Precautions in Staining of PBF

1. *Dark blue blood film:* It can be due to overstaining, inadequate washing or improper pH of the buffer. In this, RBCs are blue, nuclear chromatin is black, granules of the neutrophils are overstained and granules of the eosinophils are blue or grey.

2. *Light pink blood film:* In this, RBCs are bright red, the nuclear chromatin is pale blue and granules of the eosinophils are dark red. It can be due to understaining, prolonged washing, mounting the film before drying and improper pH of the buffer.

3. *Precipitate on the blood film:* This could be due to inadequate filtration of the stain, dust on the slide, drying during staining and inadequate washing.

Exercise 11

Differential Leucocyte Count (DLC)

Objectives

- ⇨ Discuss the method of examination of blood film for DLC and morphologic features of mature leucocytes.
- ⇨ What are the various techniques for DLC?
- ⇨ List various conditions producing variations in mature leucocytes in diseases.

EXAMINATION OF PBF FOR DLC

Choose an area near the junction of body with the tail of the smear where there is slight overlapping of RBCs i.e. neither rouleaux formation which occurs in head and body, nor totally scattered RBCs as occurs at the tail. By moving the slide in horizontal directions under oil immersion (Fig. 11.1), start counting the types of WBCs and go on entering P, L, M, E, B in a box having 100 cubes as shown in Figure 11.2. Alternatively, 100 leucocytes can be counted by pressing the keys of the automated DLC counter (Fig. 11.3). Zigzag counting of WBCs is discouraged. WBCs are then expressed as percent in the following sequence: polymorphonuclear leucocytes (P), lymphocytes (L), monocytes (M), eosinophils (E), basophils (B) i.e. P, L, M, E, B. Invariably, normal range is expressed alongside the results (Table 11.1).

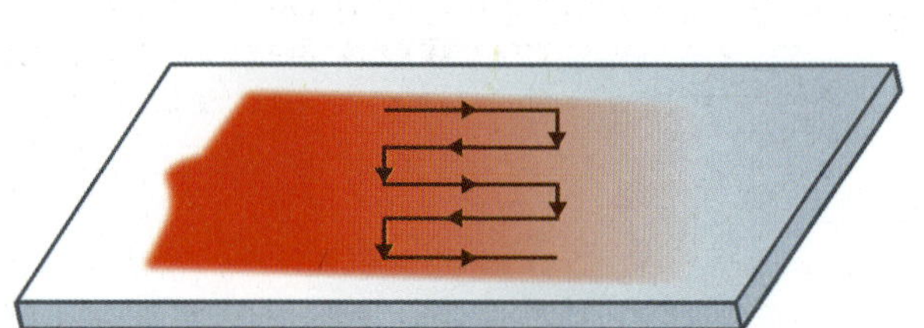

FIGURE 11.1: Counting of cells in PBF by moving in horizontal direction at the junction of the body with the tail of PBF.

L	P	P	L	P	L	P	P	L	P
P	L	P	P	L	P	P	L	P	P
P	P	P	L	P	P	L	P	P	L
P	P	P	L	P	P	P	L	P	P
L	P	L	P	M	L	L	P	M	P
P	B	E	P	P	L	P	E	P	P
P	M	P	L	L	P	L	P	L	L
L	P	E	P	P	P	L	L	P	P
P	P	P	L	P	L	P	P	L	P
P	L	L	P	P	M	P	L	P	L

Result of DLC

P	L	M	E	B
60%	32%	4%	1%	3%

FIGURE 11.2: Counting of WBCs for DLC in squares and expressing result of DLC.

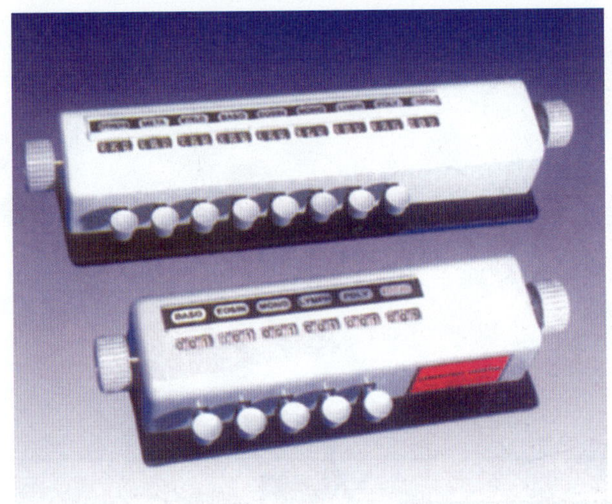

FIGURE 11.3: Counting of WBCs for DLC in DLC counters with pressing keys (Photograph by courtesy of Yorco Sales Pvt. Ltd., Delhi).

TABLE 11.1: Normal values for leucocytes in health in adults

	Normal range	*Absolute value*
Polymorphs(P)	40-75%	2,000-7,500/µl
Lymphocytes(L)	20-40%	1,500-4,000/µl
Monocytes(M)	2-10%	200-800/µl
Eosinophils(E)	1-6%	40-400/µl
Basophils(B)	0-1%	10-100/µl

MORPHOLOGIC IDENTIFICATION OF MATURE LEUCOCYTES

Polymorph (Neutrophil)

A polymorphonuclear neutrophil (PMN), commonly called polymorph or neutrophil, is 12-15 µm in diameter. It consists of a characteristic dense nucleus, having 2-5 lobes and pale cytoplasm containing numerous fine violet-pink granules.

Lymphocyte

Majority of lymphocytes in the peripheral blood are small (9-12 µm in diameter) but large lymphocytes (12-16 µm in diameter) are also found. Both small and large lymphocytes have round or slightly indented nucleus with coarsely clumped chromatin and scanty basophilic and agranular cytoplasm.

Monocyte

The monocyte is the largest mature leucocyte in the peripheral blood measuring 12-20 µm in diameter. It possesses a large, central, oval, notched or indented or horseshoe-shaped nucleus which has characteristically fine reticulated chromatin network. The cytoplasm is

TABLE 11.2: Morphology of mature leucocytes.

Feature	*Neutrophil*	*Lymphocytes (small and large)*	*Monocyte*	*Eosinophil*	*Basophil*
Morphology					
Cell diameter	12-15 µm	SL: 9-12 µm LL: 12-16 µm	12-20 µm	12-15 µm	12-15 µm
Nucleus	2-5 lobed, clumped chromatin	Large nucleus, round to indented, fills the cell, clumped chromatin	Large, lobulated, indented, with fine chromatin	Bilobed, clumped chromatin	Bilobed, clumped chromatin
Cytoplasm	Pink or violet granules	Peripheral rim of basophilic cytoplasm, no granules	Light basophilic, may contain fine granules or vacuoles	Coarse crimson red granules	Large coarse purplish granules obscuring the nucleus
Normal %	40-75	20-40	2-10	1-6	0-1
Absolute count per µl	2,000-7,500	1,500-4,000	200-800	40-400	10-100

abundant, pale blue and contains many fine granules and vacuoles.

Eosinophil

Eosinophil is similar to segmented neutrophil in size (12-15 µm in diameter) but has coarse, deep red staining granules in the cytoplasm and has usually two nuclear lobes in the form of a spectacle.

Basophil

Basophil resembles the other mature granulocytes but is distinguished by coarse, intensely basophilic granules which usually fill the cytoplasm and often overlap and obscure the nucleus.

Morphological features of different leucocytes are summarised in Table 11.2.

METHODS OF DLC

Differential leucocyte count (DLC) can be performed by two methods:

1. Visual counting
2. Automated counting

Visual Counting

This is counting of WBCs after identifying them by their morphologic features described above.

Automated Counting

It is done by electronic counting method. There are three types of electronic methods—by cell size analysis, by flow cytometry, and by high resolution pattern recognition. In addition to counting, these methods also provide additional information on cell size, shape, nuclear size and density. Automated DLC counters have a differential counting capacity of counting either 3-part DLC (granulocytes, lymphocytes and monocytes) or 5-part DLC (P, L, M, E, B). However, automated method of DLC suffers from the disadvantage that normoblasts are counted as lymphocytes and these counters are quite expensive.

PATHOLOGIC VARIATIONS IN DLC

Neutrophils

Increase in neutrophil count above 7,500/µl is called *neutrophilia* (Fig. 11.4) while fall in neutrophil count below 2,000/µl is termed neutropenia. The causes for neutrophilia and neutropenia are given in Table 11.3.

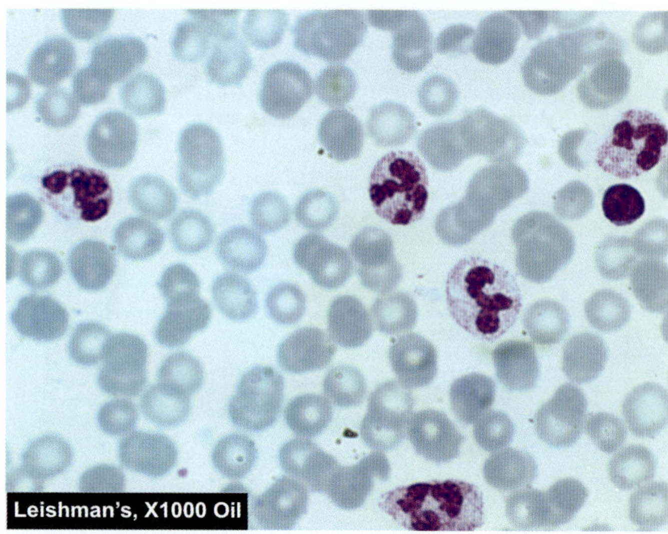

FIGURE 11.4: Neutrophilia in PBF.

TABLE 11.3: Causes of neutrophilia and neutropenia.

Neutrophilia	*Neutropenia*
1. *Acute infections*	1. *Infections*
(By bacteria, fungi,	i. Typhoid
parasites and some viruses)	ii. Brucellosis
i. Pneumonia	iii. Measles
ii. Acute appendicitis	iv. Malaria
iii. Acute cholecystitis	v. Kala azar
iv. Salpingitis	vi. Miliary tuberculosis
v. Peritonitis	2. *Drugs and chemicals*
vi. Abscess	*and physical agents*
vii. Acute tonsillitis	i. Antimetabolites
viii. Actinomycosis	ii. Benzene
ix. Poliomyelitis	iii. Nitrogen mustard
x. Furuncle	iv. Irradiation
xi. Carbuncle	3. *Haematological and*
2. *Intoxication*	*other diseases*
i. Uraemia	i. Aplastic anaemia
ii. Diabetic ketosis	ii. Pernicious
iii. Poisoning by chemicals	anaemia
iv. Eclampsia	iii. SLE
3. *Inflammation from tissue damage*	iv. Gaucher's disease
i. Burns	v. Cachexia
ii. Ischaemic necrosis	vi. Anaphylactic shock
iii. Gout	
iv. Hypersensitivity reaction	
4. *Acute haemorrhage*	
i. Acute haemolysis	
5. *Neoplastic conditions*	
i. Myeloid leukaemia (CML)	
ii. Polycythaemia vera	
iii. Myelofibrosis	
iv. Disseminated cancers	
6. *Miscellaneous conditions*	
i. Administration of corticosteroids	
ii. Idiopathic neutrophilia	

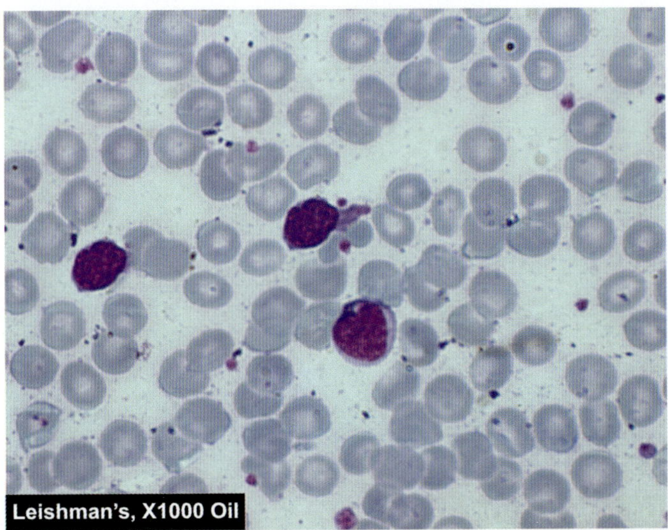

FIGURE 11.5: Lymphocytosis in PBF.

TABLE 11.4: Causes of lymphocytosis and lymphopenia.

Lymphocytosis	*Lymphopenia*
1. *Acute Infections*	i. Aplastic anaemia
i. Pertussis	ii. High dose of steroid administration
ii. Infectious mononucleosis	iii. AIDS
iii. Viral hepatitis	iv. Hodgkin's disease
2. *Chronic Infections*	v. Irradiation
i. Tuberculosis	
ii. Brucellosis	
iii. Secondary syphilis	
3. *Haematopoietic Disorders*	
i. CLL	
ii. NHL	

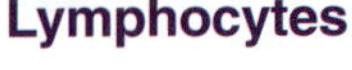

Lymphocytes

When the absolute lymphocyte count increases to more than 4,000/μl it is termed *lymphocytosis* (Fig. 11.5) while absolute lymphocyte count below 1,500/μl is called *lymphopenia;* causes for these are given in Table 11.4.

Monocytes

A rise in absolute monocyte count above 800/μl is called monocytosis (Fig. 11.6). Causes of monocytosis are given in Table 11.5.

Eosinophils

Increase in the absolute esosinophil count above 400/μl is termed *eosinophilia* (Fig. 11.7) while the fall in number is called *eosinopenia;* the causes for abnormal eosinophil count are given in Table 11.6.

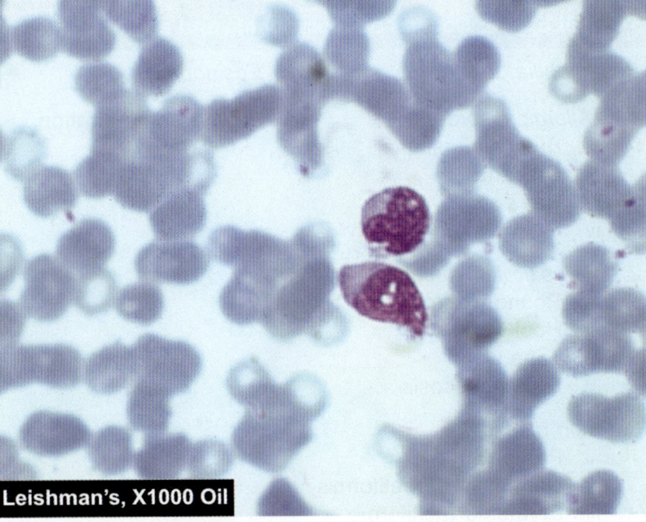

FIGURE 11.6: Monocytes in PBF.

TABLE 11.5: Monocytosis.

1. *Bacterial infections*
   - i. Tuberculosis
   - ii. SABE
   - iii. Syphilis
2. *Protozoal infections*
   - i. Malaria
   - ii. Kala azar
   - iii. Trypanosomiasis
3. *Haematopoietic disorders*
   - i. Monocytic leukaemia
   - ii. Hodgkin's disease
   - iii. Multiple myeloma
   - iv. Myeloproliferative disorders
4. *Miscellaneous conditions*
   - i. Sarcoidosis
   - ii. Cancer of ovary, breast, stomach

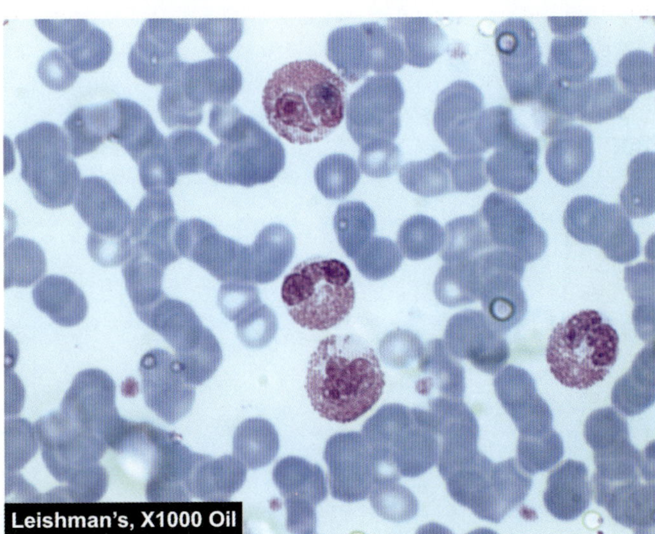

FIGURE 11.7: Eosinophilia in PBF.

TABLE 11.6: Causes of eosinophilia and eosinopenia.

Eosinophilia	*Eosinopenia*
1. *Allergic disorders* i. Bronchial asthma ii. Urticaria iii. Hay fever iv. Drug hypersensitivity	Steroid administration
2. *Parasitic infestations* i. Round worm ii. Hookworm iii. Tape worm iv. Echinococcosis	
3. *Skin diseasess* i. Pemphigus ii. Dermatitis herpetiformis iii. Erythema multiforme	
4. *Pulmonary diseases* i. Löeffler's syndrome ii. Tropical eosinophilia	
5. *Haematopoietic diseases* i. Chronic myeloid leukaemia ii. Polycythaemia vera iii. Hodgkin's disease iv. Pernicious anaemia	
6. *Miscellaneous conditions* i. Rheumatoid arthritis ii. Polyarteritis nodosa iii. Sarcoidosis iv. Irradiation	

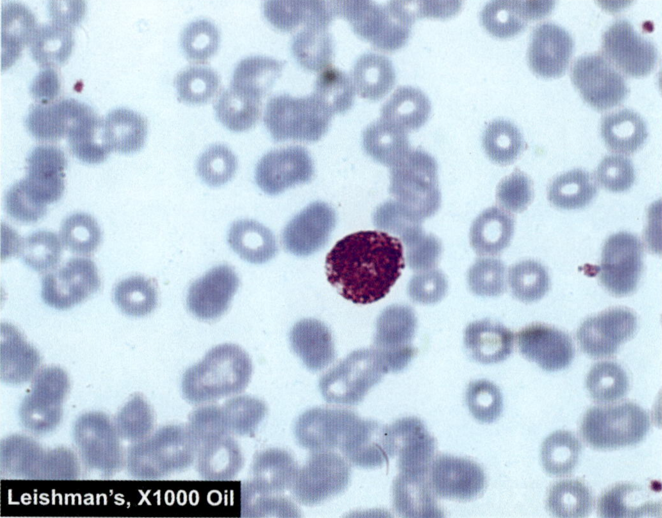

FIGURE 11.8: Basophil in PBF.

TABLE 11.7: Basophilia.

i. Chronic myeloid leukemia
ii. Polycythaemia vera
iii. Myxoedema
iv. Ulcerative colitis
v. Hodgkin's disease
vi Urticaria pigmentosa

Basophil

Basophilia refers to an increase in the absolute basophil count above 100/µl (Fig. 11.8). Causes of basophilia are given in Table 11.7.

Exercise 12

ESR, PCV (Haematocrit) and Absolute Values

Objectives

- Discuss the principle, technique and interpretation of erythrocyte sedimentation rate (ESR) and packed cell volume (PCV or haematocrit).
- How do we find absolute haematological values and what is their significance?

ERYTHROCYTE SEDIMENTATION RATE (ESR)

ESR is used as an index for presence of an active disease which could be due to many causes.

Principle

When well mixed anticoagulated blood is placed in a vertical tube, the erythrocytes tend to fall towards the bottom of the tube/pipette till they form a packed column in the lower part of the tube in a given time.

Mechanism of ESR

Fall of RBCs depends upon following factors:

i. Rouleaux formation
ii. Concentration of fibrinogen in plasma
iii. Concentration of α and β globulins
iv. Length of the tube
v. Ratio of red cells to plasma
vi. Bore of the tube
vii. Position of the tube

i) Rouleaux formation The erythrocytes sediment in the tube/pipette because their density is greater than that of plasma. When a number of erythrocytes aggregate in the form of rouleaux and settle down, their area is much less than that of the sum of the area of constituent corpuscles. The rouleaux formation is very important factor which increases the ESR.

ii) Concentration of fibrinogen It leads to colloidal changes in plasma which cause increased viscosity of plasma. Concentration of fibrinogen parallels ESR. If concentration of fibrinogen is raised, ESR is increased. In defibrinated blood, ESR is very low.

iii) Concentration of α and β globulins These protein molecules have a greater effect than other proteins in decreasing the negative charge of the RBCs that tends to keep them apart thus promoting rouleaux formation. Albumin retards the ESR; thus conditions where albumin is low ESR is more.

iv) Ratio of red cells to plasma The change in the ratio of RBCs to plasma affects ESR. When plasma is more, ESR will be increased, and vice versa.

v) Length of the tube If length of the tube/pipette is more, RBCs will have to travel a longer distance and thus ESR is low than when length of the tube is short, and vice versa.

vi) Bore of the tube If bore of the tube is more the negative charge which keeps the RBCs apart will be less and ESR will be more, and vice versa.

vii) Position of the tube If the tube/pipette is not vertical, the RBCs will have to travel less distance and ESR will be more.

Phases in ESR

ESR takes place in the following 3 phases which are carried out in sequence within one hour:

- *Phase of rouleaux formation:* In the initial period of 10 minutes, the process of rouleaux formation occurs and there is little sedimentation.

- *Phase of settling:* In the next 40 minutes, settling of RBCs occurs at a constant rate.
- *Phase of packing:* In the last 10 minutes sedimentation slows and packing of the RBCs to the bottom occurs.

That is why ESR by all methods is expressed as mm first hour rather than per hour.

Methods of ESR

1. Westergren's method
2. Wintrobe's method
3. Micro ESR method
4. Automated methods

1. Westergren's Method

Owing to its simplicity this method used to be the most commonly employed standard method prior to the AIDS-era. Westergren's pipette is a straight pipette 30 cm long open at both ends with internal bore diameter of 2.5 mm and is calibrated from 0-200 mm from top to bottom (Fig. 12.1,A).

Anticoagulant Trisodium citrate ($Na_3C_6H_5O_7.2H_2O$) as 3.8 g/dl liquid anticoagulant is used. It is used in the concentration of 1:4 i.e. four parts of blood are added to one part of anticoagulant.

Procedure

- The patient is advised to come in the morning fasting (as heavy protein diet affects concentraton of plasma proteins).
- Take 1.6 ml of patient's blood and mix it with 0.4 ml of citrate anticoagulant already put in a tube. The test should be done within two hours of taking blood.
- Fill the pipette upto mark 0 with citrated blood with the help of rubber teat by vacuum filling and fix it in a rack vertically away from sun light or vibrations.
- Let it stand for one hour after which reading is taken at the upper meniscus of the RBCs.

Normal values

Males	3-5 mm 1st hour
Females	4-7 mm 1st hour

Advantages

i. It is a more sensitive method.
ii. It is easy to fill and clean the Westergren's pipette.

Disadvantages

i. Requires more amount of blood.
ii. Dilution of blood in anticoagulant affects ESR.
iii. Filling of blood by mouth pipetting should be strictly discouraged.

2. Wintrobe's Method

The Wintrobe tube is a glass tube closed at one end. The tube is 110 mm long and has an internal bore diameter of 2.5 mm. The tube is graduated on both sides : from 0 to 10 on one side and 10 to 0 cm on the other (Fig. 12.1,B).

Anticoagulants Either of the following 2 anticoagulants can be used:

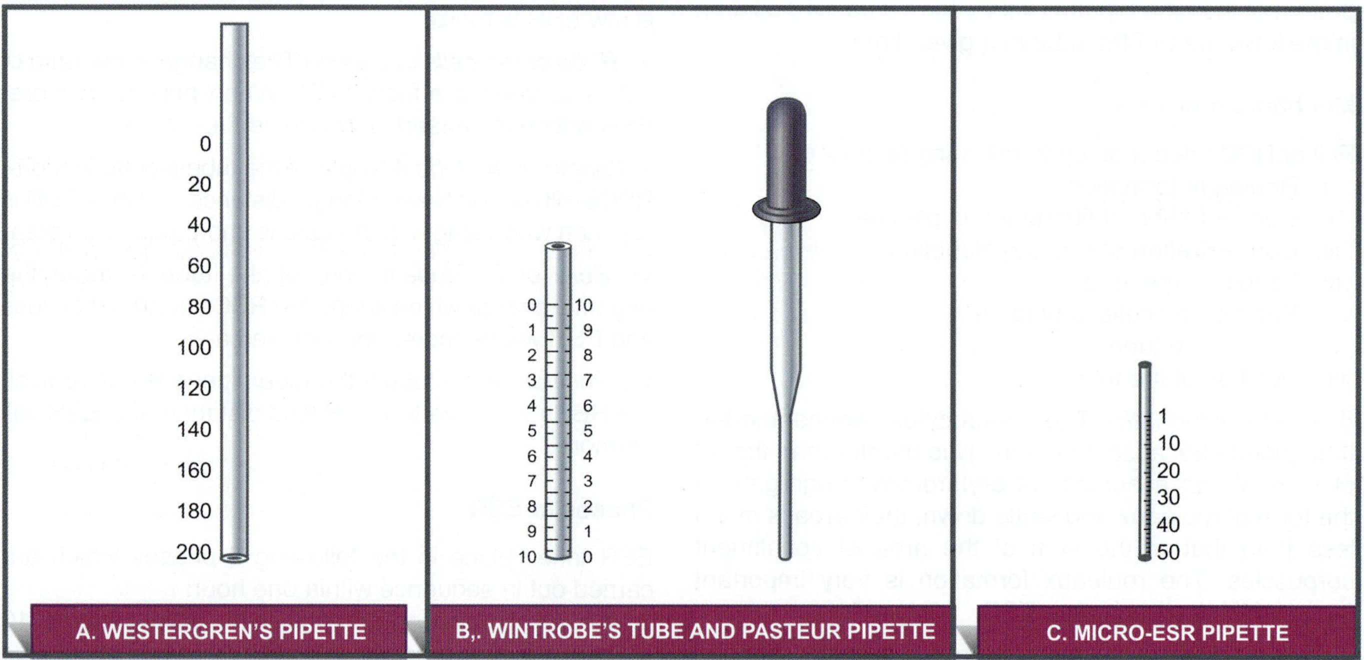

FIGURE 12.1: Westergren's pipette, Wintrobe's tube with Pasteur pipette and micro ESR pipette.

i. Ethylene diamine tetraacetic acid (EDTA) solid crystals 1-2 mg/ml.
ii. Double oxalate (solid) 2-3 mg/ml (ammonium oxalate and sodium or potassium oxalate in the ratio of 3:2; the former causes swelling and the latter causes shrinkage of RBCs and hence RBC shape is retained).

Procedure

- The patient is called in the morning fasting.
- Draw 1 ml of blood into the anticoagulant.
- Fill the Wintrobe tube upto mark 0 with anticoagulated blood with the help of a Pasteur pipette having a long stem so as to fill the tube free of air bubbles (Fig. 12.1,B).
- Place the tube vertically in a stand and note the ESR after one hour.

Normal values

Males	0-7 mm 1st hour
Females	0-15 mm 1st hour

Advantages

i. It is simple method and requires small amount of blood.
ii. There is no dilution with anticoagulant.
iii. Packed cell volume (PCV) can also be done by the same tube.
iv. Filling of tube with Pasteur pipette eliminates chance of any infection due to handling of blood.

Disadvantages

i. Because of short column and choice of anticoagulant, it is not as sensitive index of diseases.
ii. Addition of more anticoagulant can lower ESR.
iii. ESR of more than 100 mm cannot be measured.

3. Micro ESR Method

This method is used in pediatric patients or in patients where venepuncture is not possible. In this method a capillary 160 mm long with an internal bore diameter of 1 mm is used. The capillary is graduated 1 mm apart for 50 mm, with two red lines on it. Alternatively, non-graduated heparinised capillary may be used and the reading is taken by measurement of length of column (Fig. 12.1,C).

Anticoagulant Mixture of sodium citrate and EDTA is used.

Procedure

- Fill the microsedimentation pipette upto first red mark with anticoagulant.
- Fill the pipette with free flowing capillary blood upto second red mark.
- Invert it several times and allow it to stand for one hour in the sedimentation rack.
- Take the reading and results are given as that for Westergren's method.

4. Automated ESR Method

Automated closed systems use either blood collected in special evacuated tubes containing citrate or EDTA. It is taken up through a pierceable cap and then automatically diluted in the system.

Clinical Significance of ESR

ESR is a non-specific test of evaluating diseases. It is seldom used for diagnostic purpose but its use is limited to monitoring the prognosis of disease process.

Diagnostic Uses

i. Rheumatoid arthritis
ii. Chronic infections
iii. Collagen diseases
iv. Multiple myeloma
v. Macroglobulinaemia

Monitoring Prognosis of Diseases

To see the response to treatment in:

i. Tuberculosis
ii. Temporal arteritis
iii. Polymyalgia rheumatica
iv. In patients of Hodgkin's disease, ESR of < 10 mm 1st hour indicates good prognosis while ESR of > 60 mm 1st hour indicates poor prognosis.

Table 12.1 sums up the list of conditions causing raised and lowered ESR.

TABLE 12.1: Causes of abnormal ESR.

Diseases causing raised ESR	*Diseases causing low ESR*
i. Tuberculosis	i. Polycythaemia
ii. SABE	ii. Spherocytosis
iii. Acute myocardial infarction	iii. Sickle cell anaemia
	iv. Congestive heart failure
iv. Rheumatoid arthritis	v. Newborn infant
v. Shock	vi. Hypofibrinogenaemia
vi. Anaemias	
vii. Liver disease	
viii. Multiple myeloma	
ix. Pregnancy	
x. Ankylosing spondylitis	

PACKED CELL VOLUME (PCV) OR HAEMATOCRIT

PCV is defined as ratio of volume of RBCs to that of whole blood and is expressed as percentage.

Methods for Estimation of PCV

1. Macro method (Wintrobe's method)
2. Microhaematocrit method
3. Electronic method

1. Macro (Wintrobe's) Method

In this method PCV is measured by Wintrobe tube which has a length of 110 mm and internal bore of 2.5 mm and graduated from 0–10 cm on both directions. PCV by Wintrobe's method can be done on the same blood after ESR by the same tube has been done.

Procedure

- Fill the Wintrobe tube upto mark 10 with well mixed anticoagulated blood (EDTA) by Pasteur's pipette free of air bubbles.
- Centrifuge the tube at 2000-2300 g for 30 minutes.
- After centrifugation layers are noted in the wintrobe tube as under (Fig. 12.2):
  i. Uppermost layer of *plasma.*
  ii. Thin white layer of *platelets.*
  iii. Greyish-pink layer of *leucocytes.*
  iv. Lowermost is the layer of *RBCs.*
  v. Grey-white layer of leucocytes and platelets interposed between plasma above and packed RBCs below is called *buffy coat.*

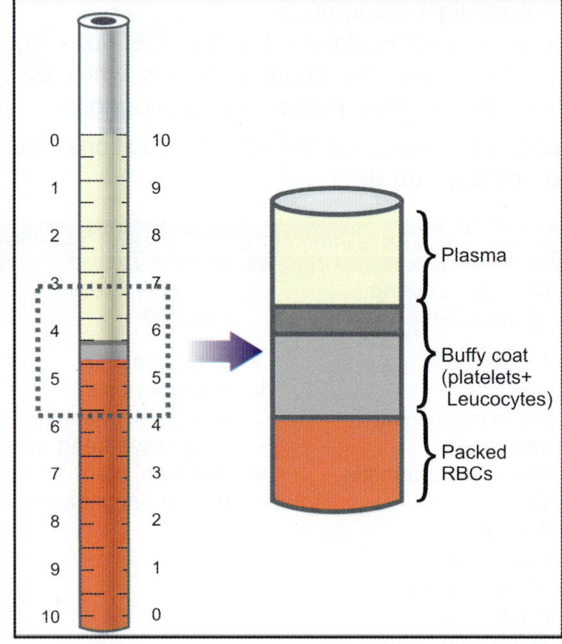

FIGURE 12.2: Haematocrit by Wintrobe's tube method.

- Note the lowermost height of column of packed RBC layer and express it as percentage.

Advantages of Macro Method

i. PCV and ESR can be measured simultaneously.
ii. Buffy coat can be prepared for other tests.
iii. By seeing the colour of plasma we can know about some of the pathological conditions e.g. in jaundice it is yellow, in haemolysis it is pink, in hyperlipidaemia it is milky.

2. Microhaematocrit Method

In this method a capillary tube 70 mm long with an internal bore of 1 mm is used and blood from skin puncture is directly taken into heparinised capillary tube.

Procedure

- Take a heparinised capillary tube.
- Fill it with blood by capillary action leaving 10 mm unfilled.
- Seal the empty end by plastic seal or by heating on flame.
- Centrifuge it in microhaematocrit centrifuge at 10,000 g for 5 minutes (Fig. 12.3).
- Measure the blood column by using a reading device which is usually a part of centrifuge.

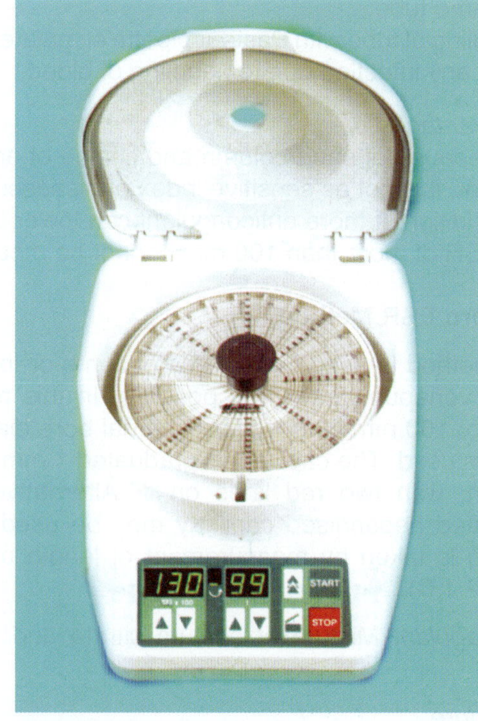

FIGURE 12.3: Microhaematocrit method for PCV. Haematocrit 20 model (Photograph courtesy of Hetlich, Germany through Global Medical System, Delhi).

TABLE 12.2: Causes of abnormal PCV.

Diseases causing raised PCV	*Diseases causing low PCV*
i. Polycythaemia	i. Anaemia
ii. Dehydration due to severe vomitings, diarrhoea, profuse sweating	ii. Pregnancy
iii. Burns	
iv. Shock	

Advantages of Micro Method

i. Less amount of blood is required.
ii. Results are available within 5 minutes.
iii. Method is more accurate, trapping of plasma is less.

Sources of Errors in Macro and Micro Methods

i. Improper handling of sample.
ii. Calibration error.
iii. Unclean and contaminated tube.
iv. Improper centrifugation time.

3. Electronic Method

Electronic methods employ automated counters where derivation of RBC count, PCV and MCV are closely interrelated.

Clinical Significance of PCV

PCV reflects the concentration of red cells and not the total red cell mass. PCV is generally three times the haemoglobin value. Table 12.2 lists the conditions causing raised and lowered PCV.

ABSOLUTE VALUES

Based on normal values of RBC count, haemoglobin and PCV, a series of absolute values or red cell indices can be derived which have diagnostic importance in various haematologic disorders. These are as under:

1. Mean corpuscular volume (MCV)

$$= \frac{\text{PCV in L/L}}{\text{RBC count/L}}$$

The normal value is 85 ± 8 fl (77-93 fl).

2. Mean corpuscular haemoglobin (MCH)

$$= \frac{\text{Hb/L}}{\text{RBC count/L}}$$

The normal range is 29.5 ± 2.5 pg (27-32 pg).

3. Mean corpuscular haemoglobin concentration (MCHC)

$$= \frac{\text{Hb/dl}}{\text{PCV in L/L}}$$

The normal value is 32.5 ± 2.5 g/dl (30-35 g/dl).

Since MCHC is independent of red cell count and size, it is considered to be of greater clinical significance as compared with other absolute values. It is low in iron deficiency anaemia but is usually normal in macrocytic anaemia.

Significance

1. In iron deficiency and thalassaemia, MCV, MCH and MCHC are reduced.
2. In anaemia due to acute blood loss and haemolytic anaemias, MCV, MCH and MCHC are all within normal limits.
3. In megaloblastic anaemias, MCV is raised above the normal range.

Exercise 13

Screening Tests for Bleeding Disorders

Objective

⇨ Discuss the principle, technique and interpretation of bleeding time (BT) and clotting time (CT).

For the investigation of a case of bleeding disorder, clinical history is very important. An accurate clinical and family history will often give an important time-saving clue to the nature of underlying bleeding disorder.

- Appearance of purpuric spots or bruises over minimally injured surface suggests an abnormality of the vascular wall.
- Continuous bleeding from mucous membranes, cuts, wounds, deeper haematomas or bleeding into the joints will suggest a defect in the blood coagulation system.
- Excessive bleeding following delivery, or retention of dead foetus, or oozing following extensive surgery, suggest the possibility of fibrinogen depletion or presence of circulating anticoagulant agents.
- History should also be taken about the ingestion of antiplatelet drugs such as aspirin.

Two of the commonly used screening tests, bleeding time (as a screening test of bleeding from platelet disorders) and whole blood clotting time (as a screening test bleeding from coagulation disorders), are discussed below.

BLEEDING TIME

Bleeding time is duration of bleeding from a standard puncture wound on the skin which is a *measure of the function of the platelets as well as integrity of the vessel wall.* This is one of the most important preliminary indicators for detection of bleeding disorders. This is also the most commonly done preoperative investigation in patients scheduled for surgery.

Principle

A small puncture is made on the skin and the time for which it bleeds is noted. Bleeding stops when platelet plug forms and breach in the vessel wall has sealed.

Methods for Bleeding Time

1. Finger tip method
2. Duke's method
3. Ivy's method

1. Finger Tip Method

Procedure

- Clean the tip of a finger with spirit.
- Prick with a disposable needle or lancet.
- Start the stop-watch immediately.
- Start gently touching the pricked finger with a filter paper till blood spots continue to be made on the filter paper.
- Stop the watch when no more blood spot comes on the filter paper and note the time.

Disadvantages

i. It is a crude method.
ii. Bleeding time is low by this method.

Normal bleeding time 1-3 minutes.

2. Duke's Method

Procedure

- Clean the lobe of a ear with a spirit swab.
- Using a disposable lancet/needle, puncture the lower edge of the earlobe to a depth of approximately 3 mm.
- Start the stop-watch immediately.
- Allow the drops of blood to fall on a filter paper without touching the earlobe and then slowly touching the blood drop gently on a new area on the filter paper.
- Stop the watch when no more blood comes over the filter paper and note the time.

Advantages of the method

i. The ear lobule has abundant subcutaneous tissue and is vascular.
ii. Flow of blood is quite good.

Normal bleeding time 3-5 minutes.

3. Ivy's Method

Procedure

- Tie the BP apparatus cuff around the patient's upper arm and inflate it upto 40 mmHg which is maintained throughout the test.
- Clean an area with spirit over the flexor surface of forearm and allow it dry.
- Using a disposable lancet or surgical blade make 2 punctures 3 mm deep 5-10 cm from each other taking care not to puncture the superficial veins.
- Start the stop-watch immediately.
- Go on blotting each puncture with a filter paper as in Duke's method.
- Stop the watch, note the time in each puncture and calculate average bleeding time (Fig. 13.1).

Advantages of the method

i. This is the method of choice.
ii. It is a standardised method.
iii. Bleeding time is more accurate.

Normal bleeding time 3-8 minutes.

Clinical Application of Bleeding Time

The bleeding time is *prolonged* in:

i. Thrombocytopenia
ii. Disorders of platelet functions
iii. Acute leukaemias
iv. Aplastic anaemias
v. Liver disease
vi. von Willebrand's disease
vii. DIC
viii. Abnormalilty in the wall of blood vessels
ix. Administration of drugs prior to test e.g. aspirin

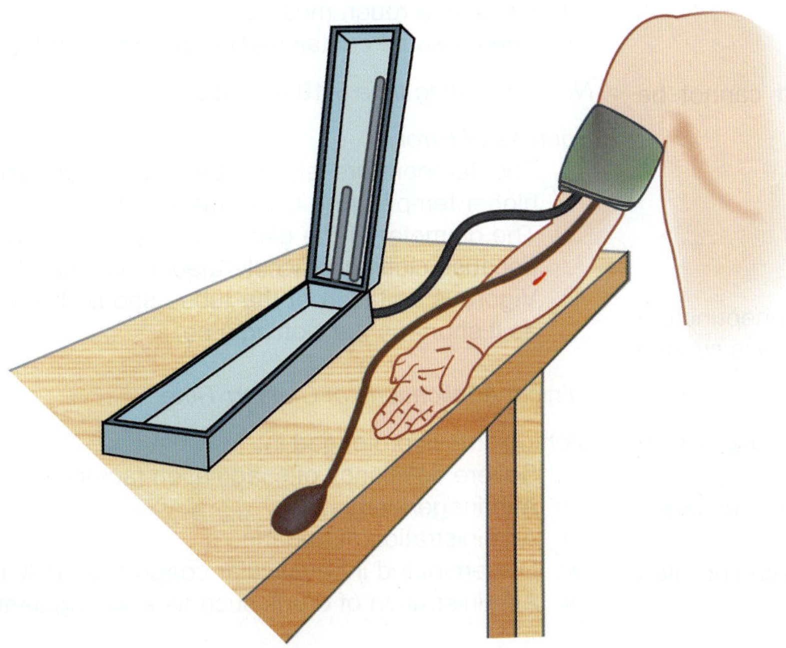

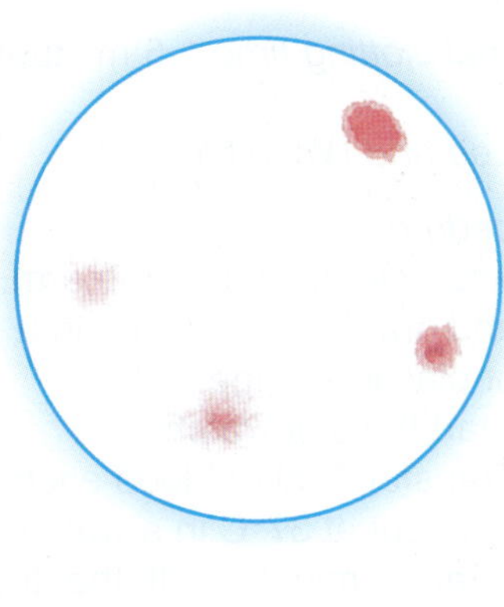

FIGURE 13.1: Ivy's method for bleeding time.

CLOTTING TIME

This is also known as whole blood clotting time and is a *measure of the plasma clotting factors.* It is a screening test for coagulation disorders.

Various other tests for coagulation disorders include: prothrombin time (PT), partial thromboplastin time (PTTK) or activated partial thromboplastin time with kaolin (APTTK), and measurement of fibrinogen.

There are two methods of whole blood clotting time:

1. Capillary tube method
2. Lee and White method

1. Capillary Tube Method

Procedure

- Clean the tip of a finger with spirit.
- Puncture it upto 3 mm deep with a disposable needle.
- Start the stopwatch.
- Fill two capillary tubes with free flowing blood from the puncture after wiping the first drop of blood.
- Keep these tubes at body temperature.
- After 2 minutes, start breaking the capillary tube at 1 cm distance to see whether a thin fibrin strand is formed between the two broken ends.
- Stop the watch and calculate the time from average of the two capillary tubes.

Disadvantages

i. Method is insensitive.
ii. Method is unreliable.

Advantages

It can be performed when venous blood cannot be obtained.

Normal clotting time 1-5 mintues.

2. Lee and White Method

Procedure

- After cleaning the forearm, make a venepuncture and draw 3 ml of blood in a siliconised glass syringe or plastic syringe.
- Start the stopwatch.
- Transfer 1 ml of blood each into 3 glass tubes which are kept at 37°C in a waterbath (Fig. 13.2).
- After 3 minutes tilt the tubes one by one every 30 seconds.
- The clotting time is taken when the tubes can be tilted without spilling of their contents.

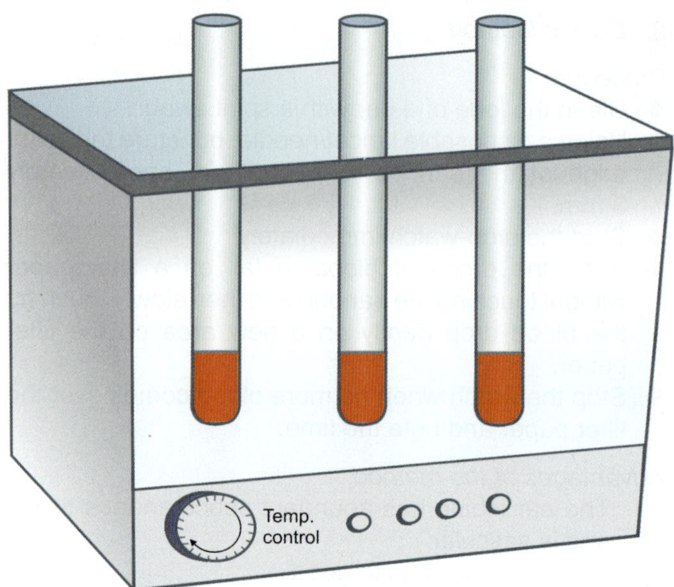

FIGURE 13.2: Lee and White method for clotting time.

- Calculate the clotting time by average of 3 tubes.

Advantages

i. More accurate and standard method.
ii. Test can be run with control.

Disadvantages

i. It is also a rough method.
ii. There can be contamination of syringe or tubes.

Normal clotting time 5-10 mintues.

Sources of Error

i. The temperature should be maintained because higher temperature accelerates clotting.
ii. The diameter of the glass tubes should be uniform because clotting is accelerated in narrow tubes.
iii. Vigorous agitation of the tubes should be avoided as it shortens the clotting time.

Clinical Applications of Clotting Time

Clotting time is prolonged in:

i. Severe deficiency of coagulation factors.
ii. Afibrinogenaemia.
iii. Administration of heparin.
iv. Disseminated intravascular coagulation (DIC).
v. Administration of drugs such as anticoagulants.

Section Four

HISTOPATHOLOGY

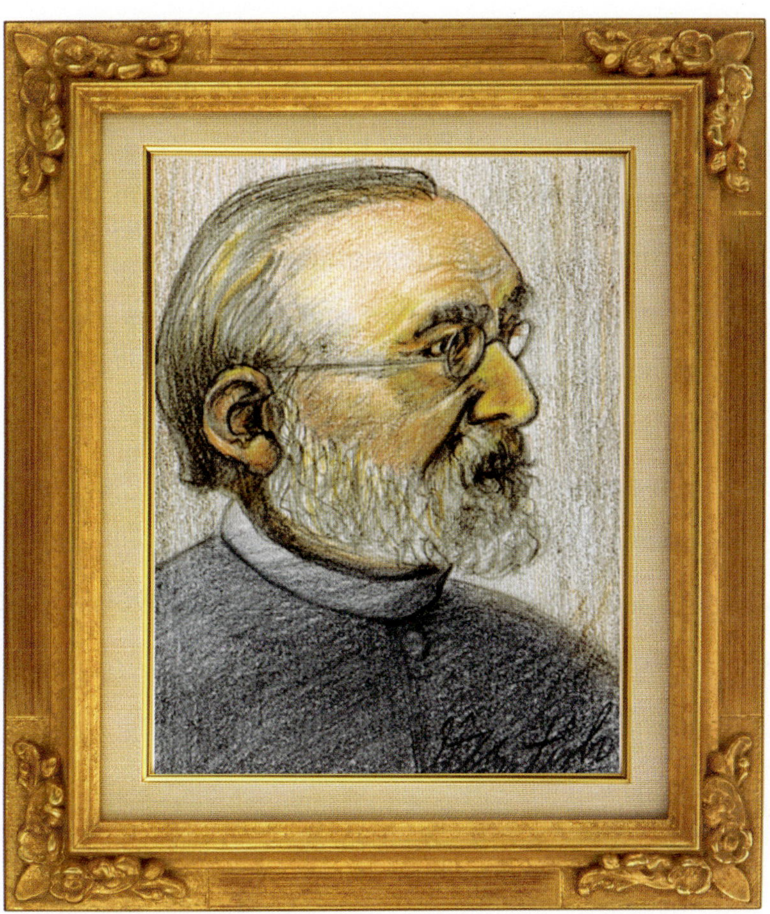

RUDOLF VIRCHOW (1821–1902)
'FATHER OF MODERN PATHOLOGY'

German physician, who described cellular basis of disease and introduced histopathology as a diagnostic branch. Important discoveries going by his name include: Virchow cells (lepra cell), Virchow node (enlarged left supraclavicular lymph node in cancer of the stomach), Virchow space in brain tissue, and Virchow's triad in pathogenesis of thrombosis.

Section Contents

Exercise

14

Degenerations and Necrosis

Objectives

- ⇨ Learn common forms of degenerations and necrosis with one example each—hyaline change (e.g. leiomyoma), coagulative necrosis (e.g. infarct kidney) and liquefactive necrosis (e.g. infarct brain)*.
- ⇨ Describe salient gross and microscopic features of these conditions.

HYALINE CHANGE IN LEIOMYOMA

The word hyaline simply refer to morphologic appearance of the material that has glassy, pink, homogeneous appearance when routinely stained with haematoxylin and eosin. Hyaline change (or hyalinisation) represents an endstage of many diverse and unrelated lesions. It may be intracellular or extracellular. Hyaline degeneration in leiomyoma, a benign smooth muscle tumour, is an example of extracellular hyaline in the connective tissue. Uterine leiomyomas may be subserosal, intramural or submucosal.

G/A The tumour is circumscribed, firm to hard. Cut surface presents a whorled appearance. The hyalinised area in the tumour appears glassy and homogeneous (Fig. 14.1).

M/E

i. There is mixture of smooth muscle fibres and fibrous tissue in varying proportions. Some of the muscle fibres may be cut longitudinally and some transversely.
ii. Smooth muscle fibres admixed with fibrous tissue are arranged in a whorled pattern at many places.
iii. Nuclei of the smooth muscle fibres are short, plump and fusiform while those of the fibroblasts are longer, slender and curved
iv. Hyaline degeneration which is the commonest change due to insufficient blood supply appears as pink, homogeneous and acellular material (Fig. 14.2).

COAGULATIVE NECROSIS (INFARCT) KIDNEY

Coagulative necrosis is the most common type of necrosis caused by irreversible focal cell injury, most often from sudden cessation of blood supply or ischaemia (infarction). The characteristic examples of coagulative necrosis are seen in infarcts of the kidney and spleen, resulting from thromboemboli.

G/A Renal infarcts are often multiple and may be bilateral. Characteristically, they are pale or anaemic and wedge-shaped with base resting under the capsule and apex pointing towards the medulla. Generally, a narrow rim of renal tissue under the capsule is spared because it draws its blood supply from the capsular vessels. The cut surface of renal infarct in the initial 2 to 3 days is red and congested but by 4th day the centre becomes pale

*Caseous necrosis is discussed later in Exercise 18.

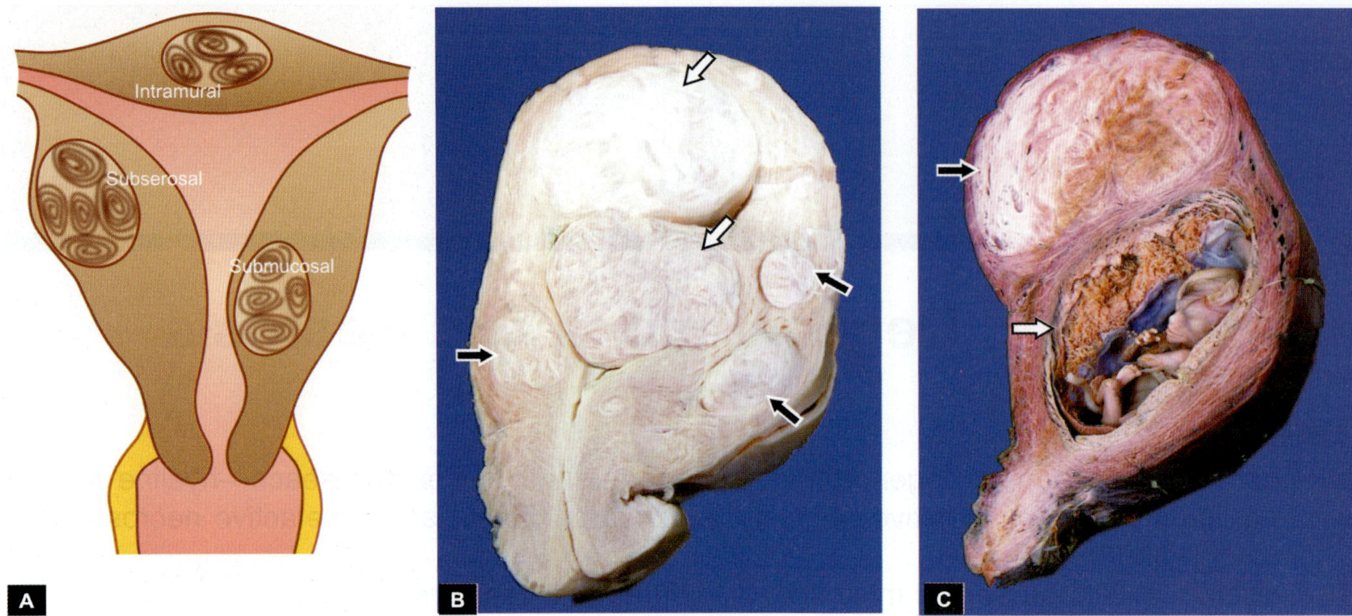

FIGURE 14.1: Leiomyomas uterus. A, Diagrammatic appearance of common locations and characteristic whorled appearance on cut section. B, Sectioned surface of the uterus shows multiple circumscribed, firm nodular masses of variable sizes—submucosal (white arrows) and intramural (black arrows) in location having characteristic whorling. C, The opened up uterine cavity shows an intrauterine gestation sac with placenta (white arrow) and a single circumscribed, enlarged, firm nodular mass in intramural location (black arrow) having grey-white whorled pattern.

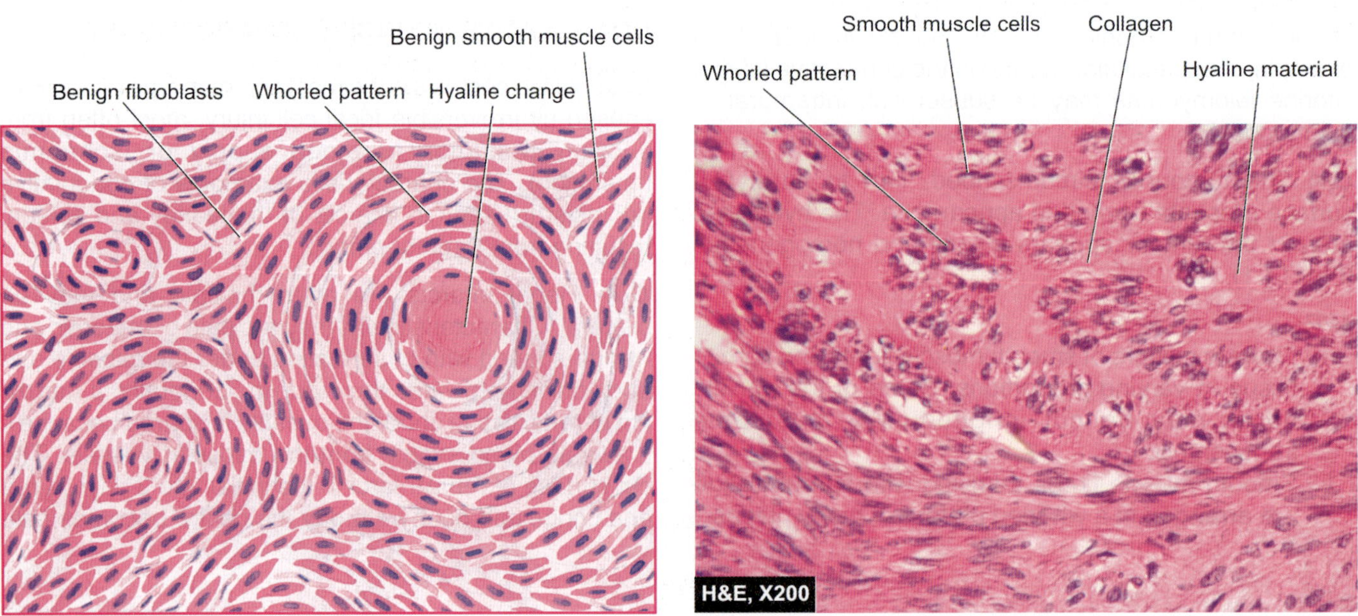

FIGURE 14.2: Leiomyomas. Microscopy shows whorls of smooth muscle cells which are spindle-shaped, having abundant cytoplasm and oval nuclei and mixed with fibrous tissue. The hyaline material appears homogeneous, pink and glassy.

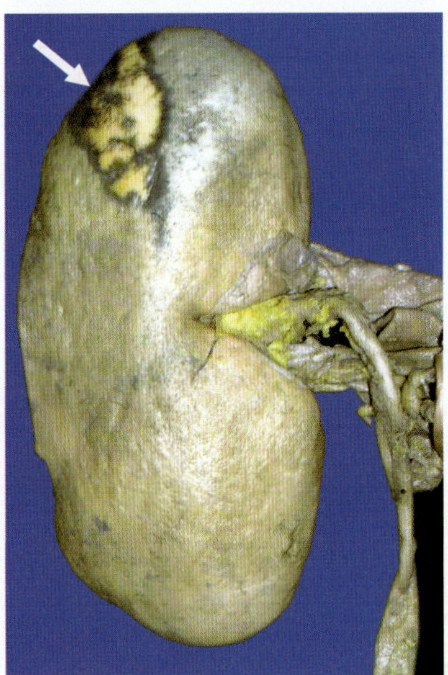

FIGURE 14.3: Infarct kidney. The wedge-shaped infarct is slightly depressed on the surface. The apex lies internally and wide base is on the surface. The central area is pale while the margin is haemorrhagic.

yellow. At the end of one week, the infarct is typically anaemic and depressed below the surface of the kidney (Fig. 14.3).

M/E

i. The hallmark of coagulative necrosis is that architectural outlines of glomeruli and tubules may be preserved though all cellular details are lost.
ii. The margin of infarct shows inflammatory reaction, initially by polymorphonuclear cells but later macrophages, lymphocytes and fibrous tissue predominate (Fig. 14.4).

LIQUEFACTIVE NECROSIS (INFARCT) BRAIN

Liquefactive necrosis results commonly due to bacterial infections which constitute powerful stimuli for release of hydrolytic enzymes causing liquefaction. The common example is infarct of the brain.

G/A The affected area of the brain is soft with liquefied centre containing necrotic debris. Later, a cyst wall is formed.

M/E

i. The cystic space contains necrotic cell debris and macrophages containing phagocytosed material.
ii. The cyst wall is formed by proliferating capillaries, inflammatory cells and proliferating glial cells (gliosis) (Fig. 14.5).

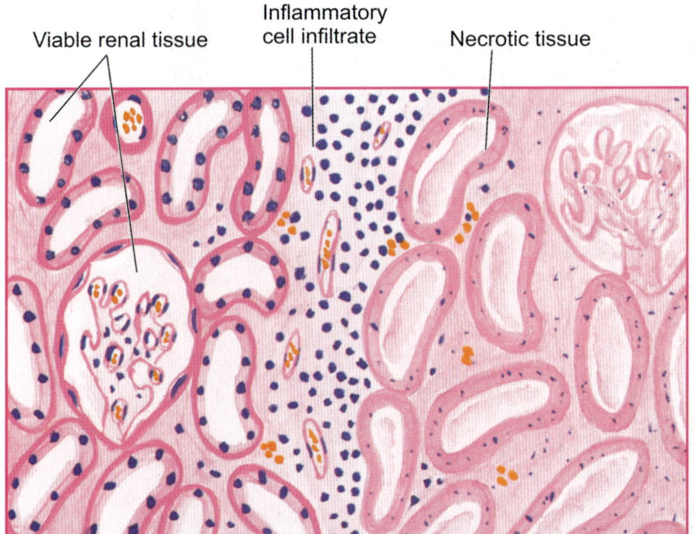

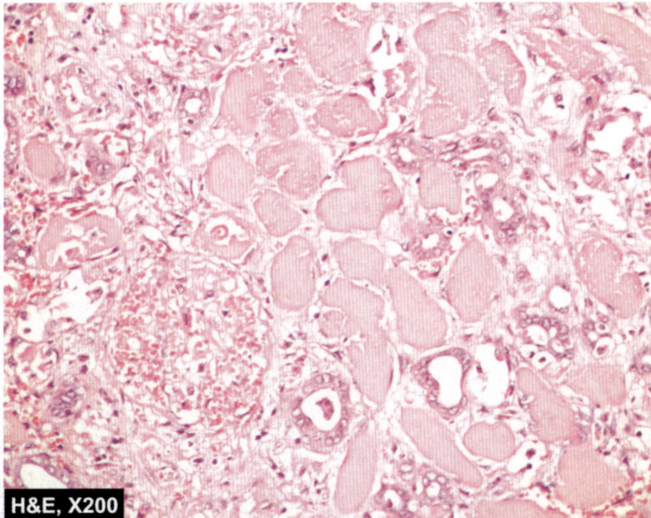

FIGURE 14.4: Coagulative necrosis in infarct kidney. The affected area on right shows cells with intensely eosinophilic cytoplasm of tubular cells but the outlines of tubules are still maintained. The nuclei show granular debris. The interface between viable and non-viable area shows non-specific chronic inflammation and proliferating vessels.

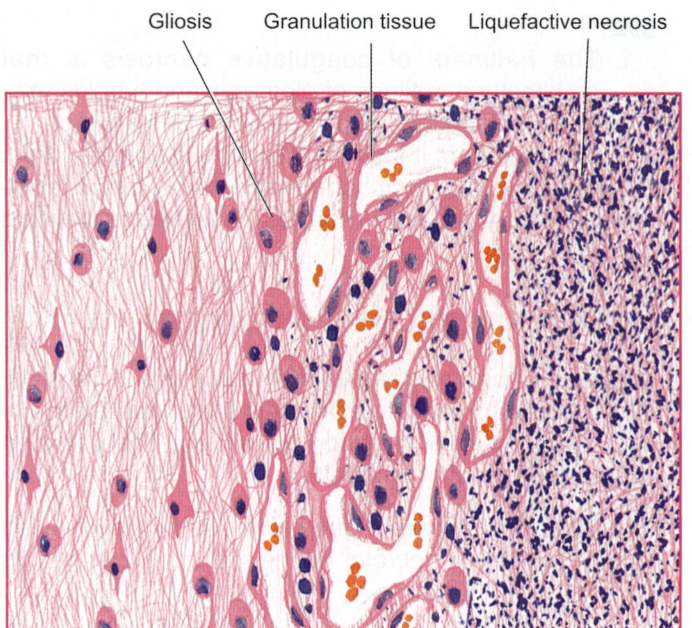

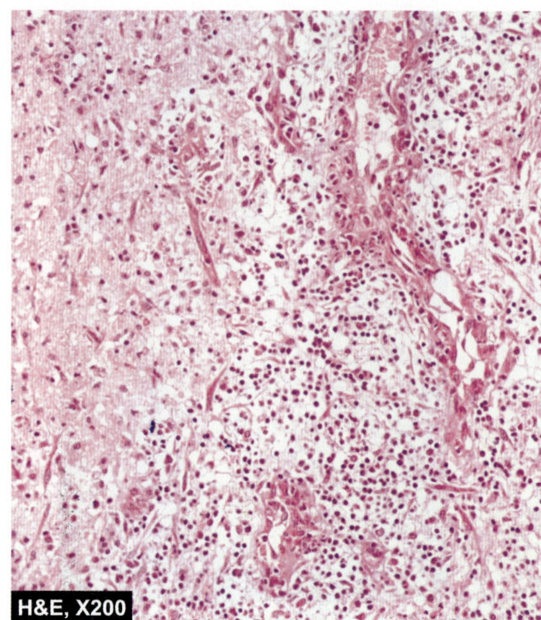

FIGURE 14.5: Liquefactive necrosis brain. The necrosed area on right side of the field shows a cystic space containing cell debris, while the surrounding zone shows granulation tissue and gliosis.

Exercise

15

Intracellular Accumulations and Amyloidosis

Objectives

- Learn common forms of intracellular accumulations and amyloidosis with examples—fat (e.g. fatty change liver), amyloid deposits (e.g. kidney, spleen).
- Describe salient gross and microscopic features of these conditions.

FATTY CHANGE LIVER

Fatty change (steatosis) is seen most commonly in the liver since it is the major organ involved in fat metabolism. The causes include alcohol abuse (most common cause in industrialised world), protein malnutrition, obesity, diabetes mellitus, anoxia, and various toxins (carbon tetrachloride, chloroform, ether, etc).

G/A The liver is enlarged and yellow with tense, glistening capsule and rounded margins. The cut surface bulges slightly and is pale-yellow and greasy to touch (Fig. 15.1).

M/E

i. Fat in the cytoplasm of the hepatocytes is seen as clear area which may vary from minute droplets in the cytoplasm of a few hepatocytes *(microvesicular)* to distention of the entire cytoplasm of most cells by coalesced droplets *(macrovesicular)* pushing the nucleus to periphery of the cell (Fig. 15.2).
ii. When the steatosis is mild, centrilobular hepatocytes are mainly affected, while the progressive accumulation of fat involves the entire lobule.
iii. Occasionally, the adjacent cells containing fat rupture producing fatty cysts.
iv. Infrequently, lipogranulomas may appear consisting of collection of macrophages, lymphocytes and multinucleate giant cells.

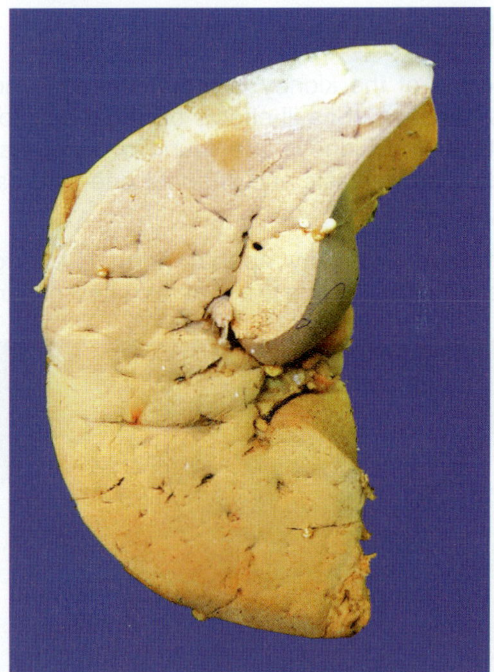

FIGURE 15.1: Fatty liver. Sectioned slice of the liver shows pale yellow parenchyma with rounded borders.

v. Special stains such as Sudan III, Sudan IV, Sudan black and oil red O can be employed to demonstrate fat in the tissue.

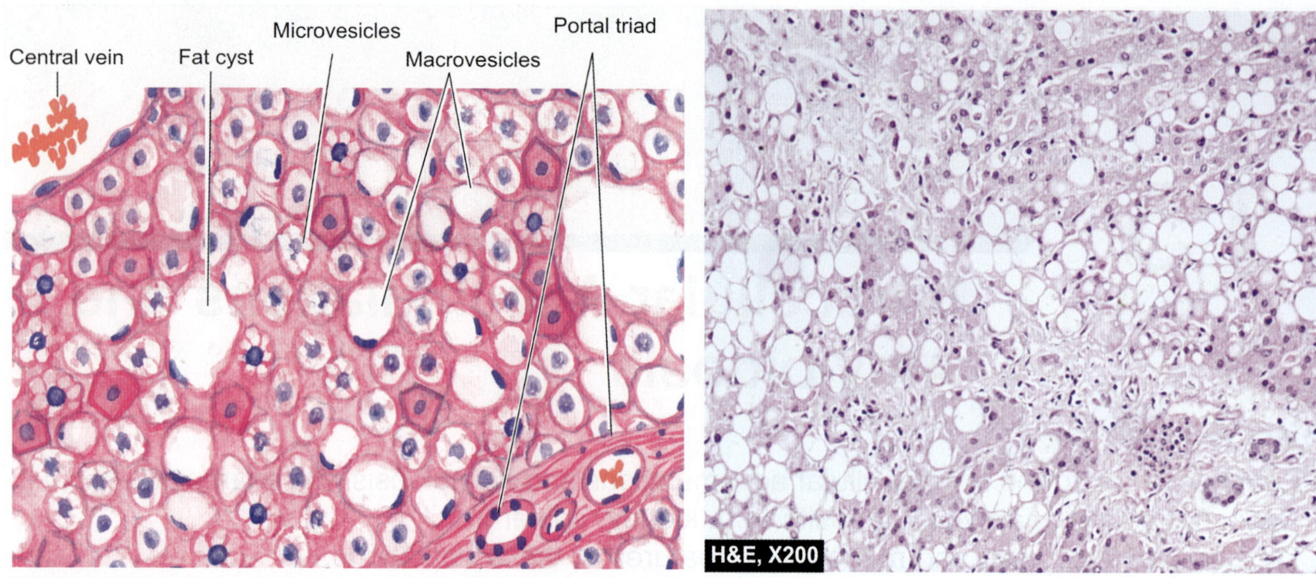

FIGURE 15.2: Fatty liver. Many of the hepatocytes are distended with large fat vacuoles pushing the nuclei to the periphery (macrovesicles), while others show multiple small vacuoles in the cytoplasm (microvesicles).

AMYLOIDOSIS KIDNEY

Amyloidosis of the kidney is most common and most serious because of its ill-effects on renal function. The deposits in the kidneys are found in most cases of secondary amyloidosis and in about one-third cases of primary amyloidosis.

G/A The kidneys may appear normal, enlarged or terminally contracted due to ischaemic effect of narrowing of vascular lumina. The cut surface is pale, waxy and translucent (Fig. 15.3).

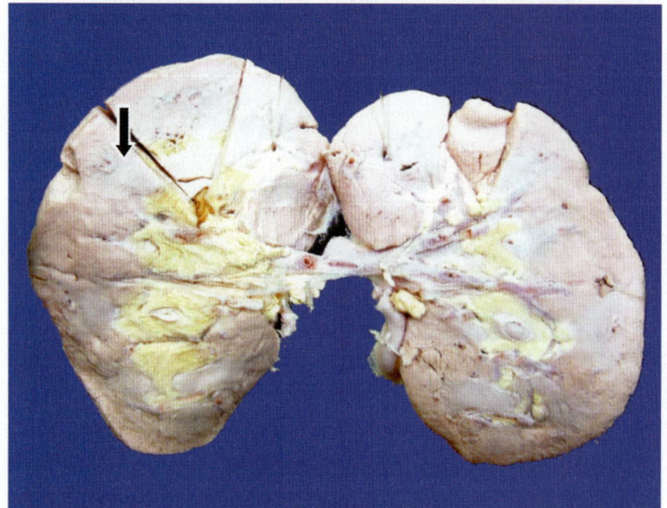

FIGURE 15.3: Amyloidosis of kidney. The kidney is small and pale in colour. Sectioned surface shows loss of corticomedullary distinction (arrow) and pale, waxy translucency.

M/E

i. The amyloid is seen as amorphous, eosinophilic, hyaline extracellular material. It is deposited mainly in the *glomeruli*, initially on the glomerular basement membrane but later extends to produce luminal narrowing and distortion of the glomerular capillary tuft.
ii. The amyloid deposits in the *tubules* begin close to the tubular epithelial basement membrane. Subsequently, the deposits may produce degenerative changes in the tubular epithelial cells and amyloid casts in the tubular lumina.
iii. The walls of small *arteries and arterioles* in the interstitium of the kidney are narrowed due to amyloid deposit (Fig. 15.4).
iv. *Congo red staining* imparts pink or red colour to the amyloid when seen in ordinary light but demonstrates green birefringence when viewed under polarising microscopy (Fig. 15.5, A, B).

AMYLOIDOSIS SPLEEN

Splenic amyloid may have two patterns—one associated primarily with deposition in the stroma of the red pulp (lardaceous spleen) and the second with in the stroma of the white pulp (sago spleen).

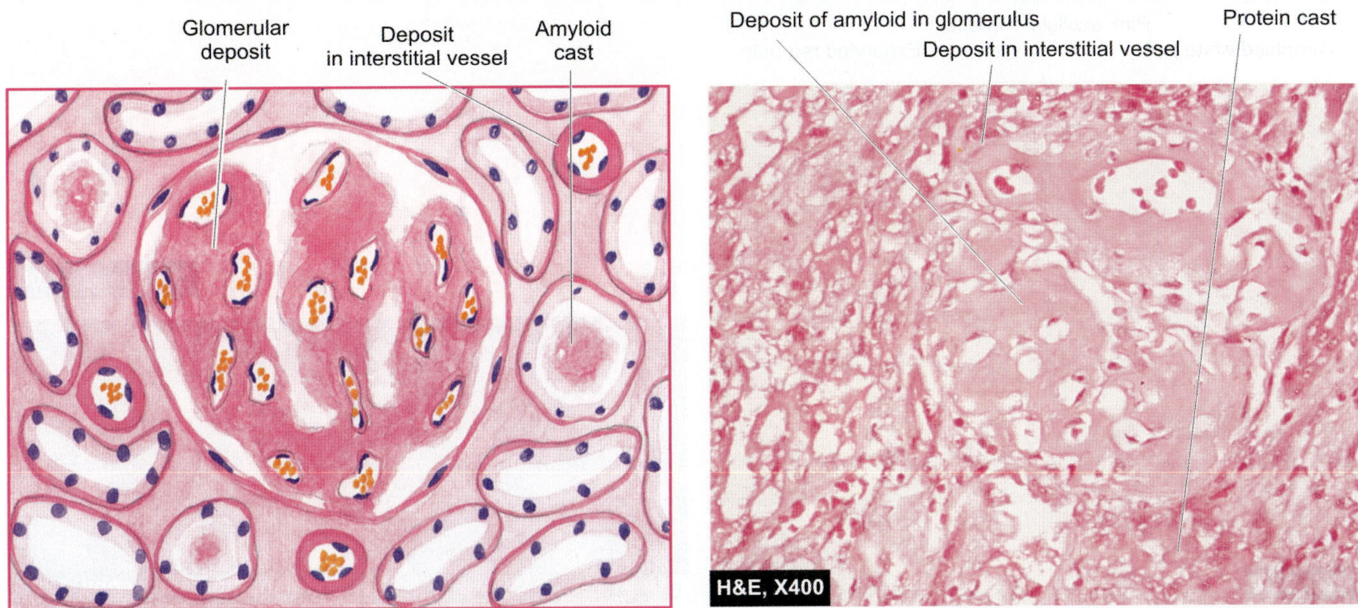

Figure 15.4: Amyloidosis of kidney. The amyloid deposits are seen mainly in the glomerular capillary tuft. The deposits are also present in peritubular connective tissue producing atrophic tubules and amyloid casts in the tubular lumina, and in the arterial wall producing luminal narrowing.

G/A The spleen may be normal-sized or may cause moderate to marked splenomegaly. The cut surface of the spleen shows one of the two patterns of deposition—*lardaceous spleen* characterised by diffuse map-like areas of pale, waxy translucency (Fig. 15.6) or, alternatively, *sago spleen* seen as multiple pale foci corresponding to the regions of splenic follicles.

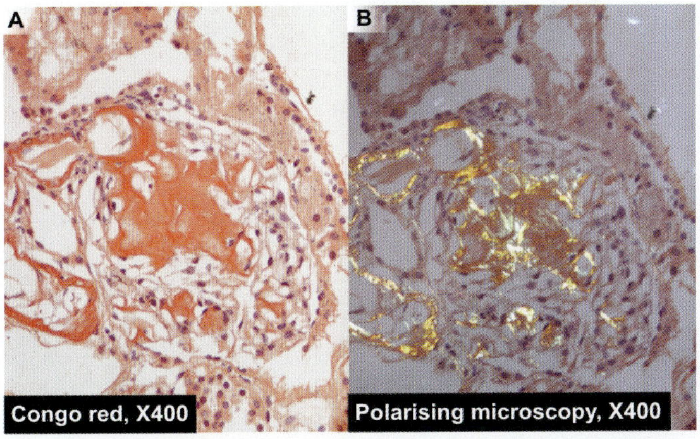

A
B
Congo red, X400
Polarising microscopy, X400

Figure 15.5: Amyloidosis kidney, Congo red stain. A, The amyloid deposits are seen mainly in the glomerular capillary tuft stained red-pink (Congophilia). B, Viewing the same under polarising microscopy, the congophilic areas show apple-green birefringence.

M/E

i. In *lardaceous spleen* the amyloid deposits are seen in the walls of splenic sinuses and the region of the red pulp.

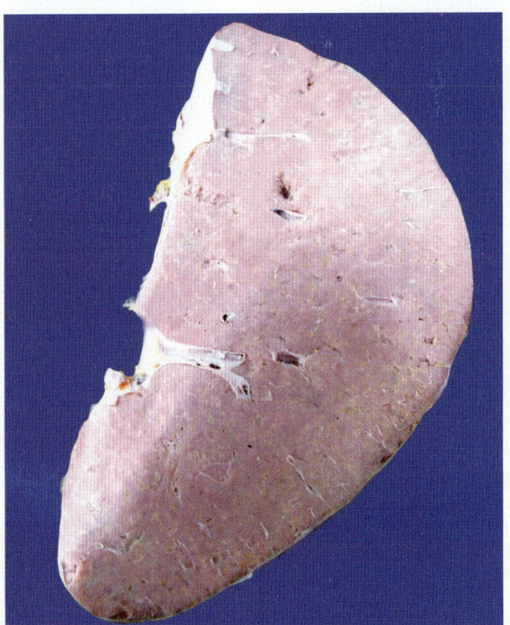

Figure 15.6: Lardaceous amyloidosis of the spleen. The sectioned surface shows presence of plae waxy translucency in a map-like pattern.

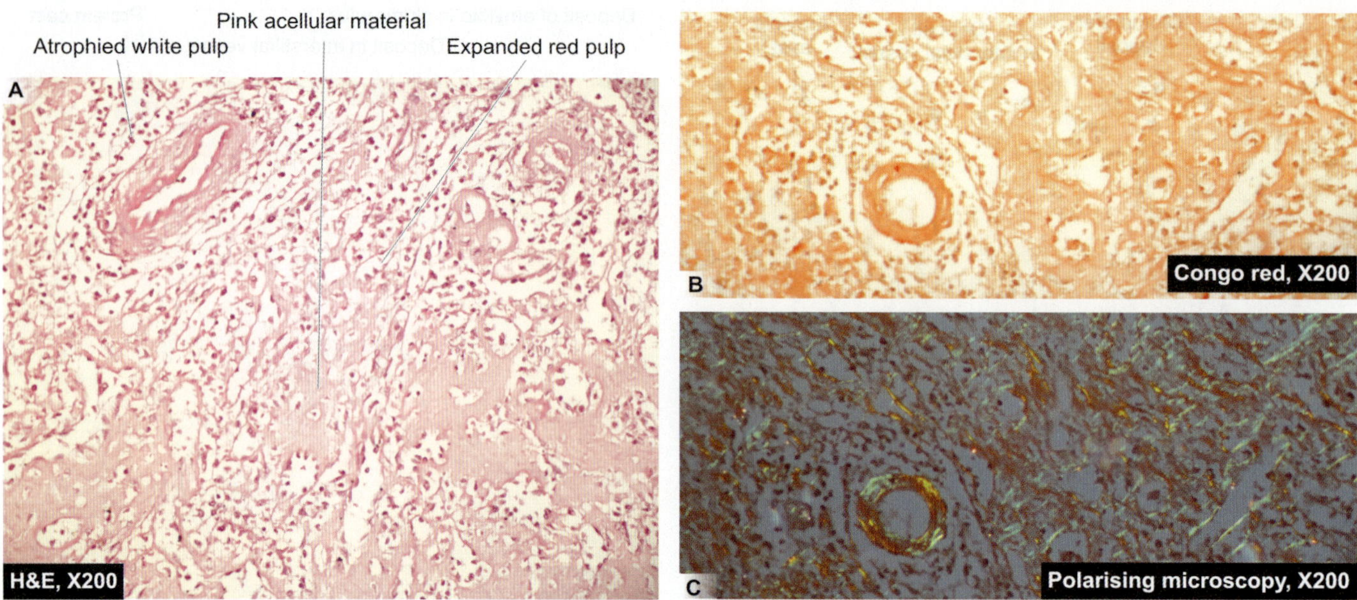

Figure 15.7: Amyloidosis spleen. A, The pink acellular amyloid material is seen in the red pulp causing atrophy of white pulp. B, Congo red staining shows Congophilia as seen by red-pink colour. C, When viewed under polarising microscopy the corresponding area shows apple-green birefringence.

ii. In *sago spleen*, the amyloid deposits begin in the walls of the arterioles of the white pulp and eventually replacing the splenic follicles (Fig. 15.7,A).

iii. *Congo red staining* gives pink or red colour to amyloid by light microscopy and when viewed in polarising light shows green birefringence (Fig. 15.7, B, C).

Exercise

16

Derangements of Body Fluids

Objectives

⇨ Learn important forms of derangements of body fluids with examples—chronic venous congestion (e.g. CVC lung, CVC liver), obstruction in circulation (e.g. thrombus artery).

⇨ Describe salient gross and microscopic features of these conditions.

CVC LUNG

Chronic venous congestion of lungs and consequent pulmonary oedema occur in elevated left atrial pressure which raises the pulmonary venous pressure e.g. in mitral stenosis in rheumatic heart disease.

G/A Both lungs are dark brown in colour, heavy and firm. Cut surface shows brown coloration referred to as *brown induration*.

M/E

i. Vessels in the alveolar septa are dilated and congested.
ii. Rupture of dilated and congested capillaries may result in minute intra-alveolar haemorrhages.
iii. The characteristic finding is the presence of large number of alveolar macrophages filled with yellow-brown haemosiderin pigment, so called *heart failure cells* in the alveoli (Fig. 16.1).

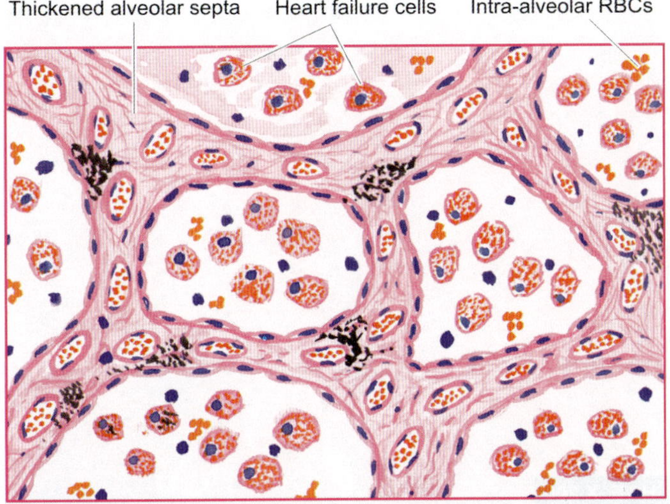

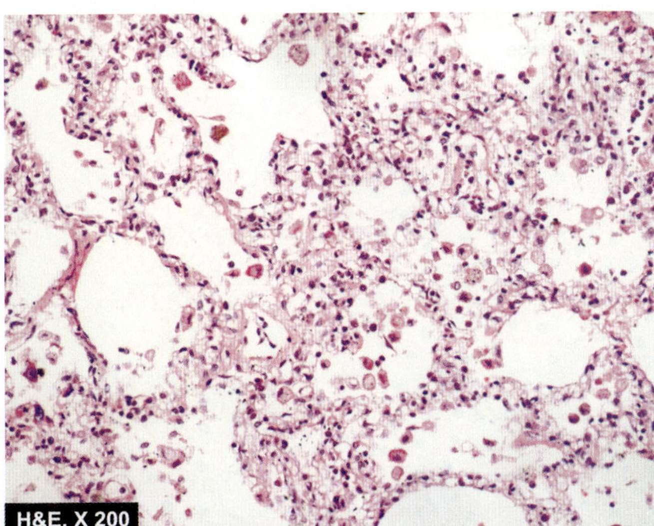

FIGURE 16.1: CVC lung. The alveolar septa are widened and thickened due to congestion, oedema and mild fibrosis. The alveolar lumina contain heart failure cells (alveolar macrophages containing haemosiderin pigment).

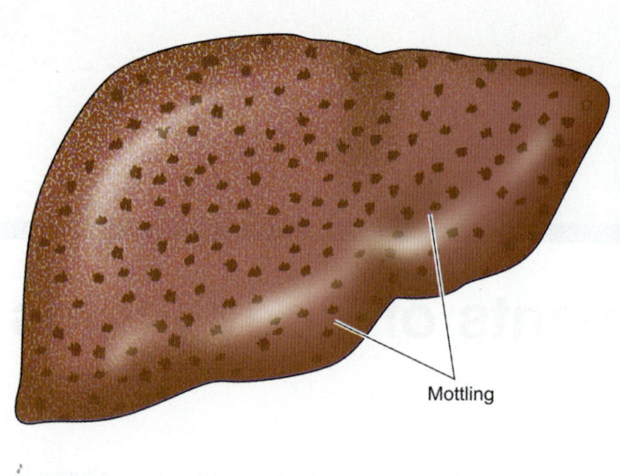

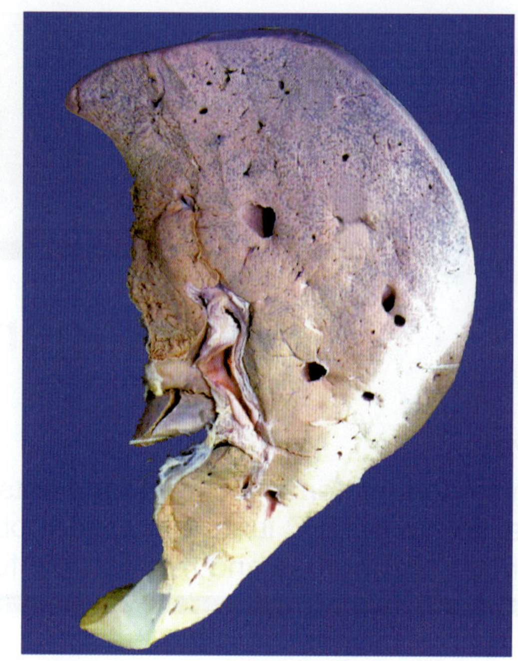

FIGURE 16.2: Nutmeg liver. The cut surface shows mottled appearance—alternate pattern of dark congestion and pale fatty change.

iv. Pulmonary oedema is a common accompaniment of venous congestion of the lungs.

CVC LIVER

The liver is particularly vulnerable to chronic passive congestion in right heart failure.

G/A The liver is enlarged and tender. The cut surface shows characteristic alternate dark areas representing congested centre of each lobule, and light areas being the fatty peripheral part, so called *nutmeg liver* (Fig. 16.2).

M/E

i. The central vein and the sinusoids in the centrilobular region are distended with blood.
ii. The hepatocytes in the centrilobular region undergo degeneration and atrophy, probably as a result of anoxia.

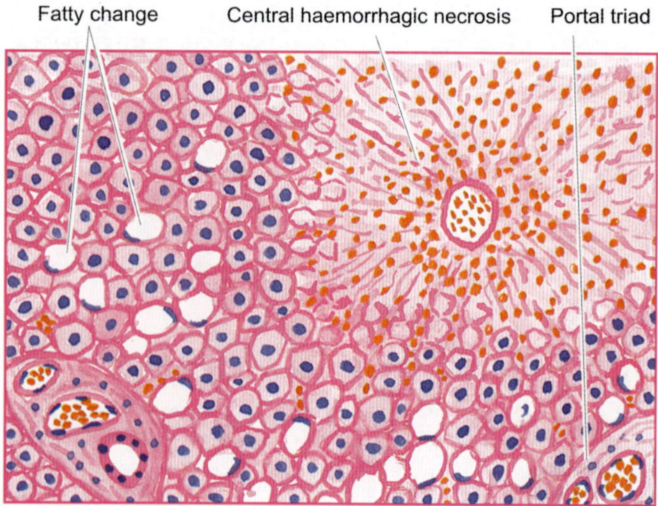

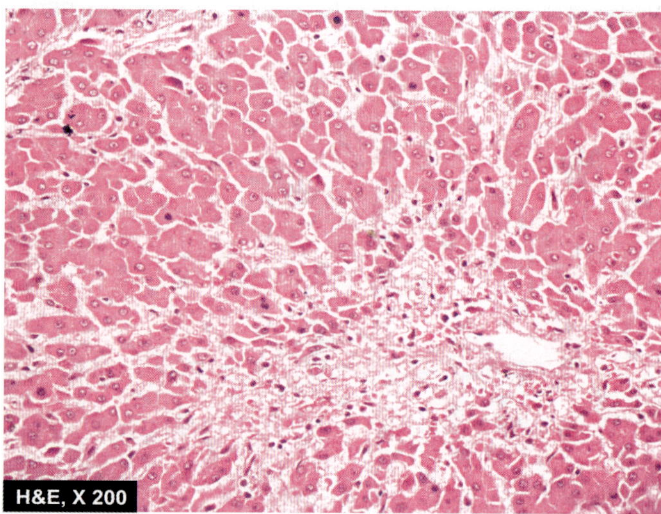

FIGURE 16.3: CVC liver. The centrilobular zone shows marked degeneration and necrosis of hepatocytes accompanied by haemorrhage while the peripheral zone shows mild fatty change of liver cells.

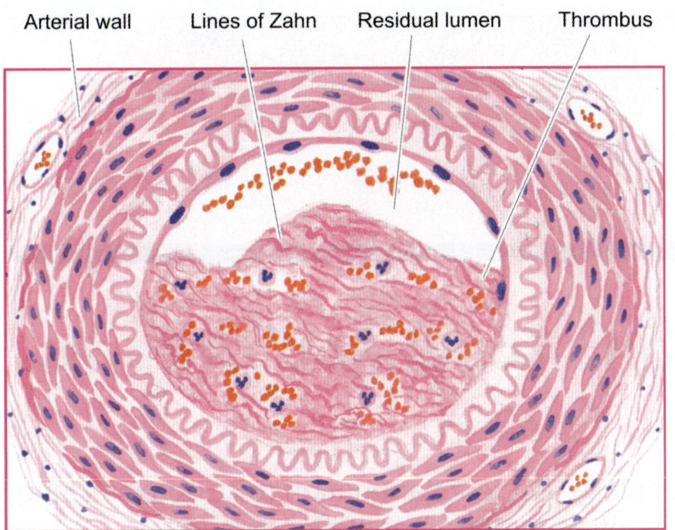

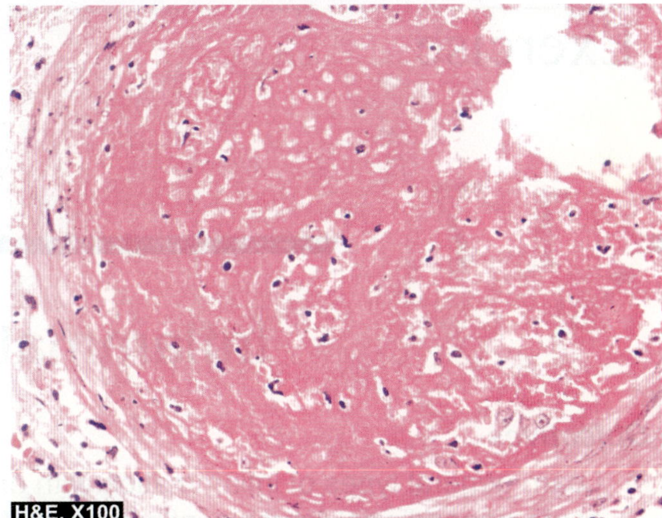

FIGURE 16.4: Thrombus in an artery. The thrombus is adherent to the arterial wall and is seen occluding most of the lumen. It shows lines of Zahn composed of granular-looking platelets and fibrin meshwork with entangled red cells and leucocytes.

iii. Eventually, the centrilobular zone shows central haemorrhagic necrosis (Fig. 16.3).
iv. The peripheral hepatocytes are either normal or may show fatty change.

THROMBUS ARTERY

Thrombi may occur anywhere in the arteries but the most common site is in the coronary arteries.

G/A Coronary arterial thrombi are generally firmly attached to the vessel wall (mural) and occlude the lumen (occlusive). The arterial thrombus invariably overlies an atherosclerotic lesion. A slit-like lumen may be formed on contraction of freshly-formed thrombus restoring some flow. Arterial thrombus is grey-white and friable. The cut surface shows laminations called the lines of Zahn.

M/E

i. The internal elastic lamina is degenerated and disrupted at the site of attachment of thrombus to the vessel wall.
ii. The residual lumen of the original artery is slit-like and shows flowing blood (Fig. 16.4).
iii. The structure of thrombus shows lines of Zahn composed of layers of light-staining fibrin strands and platelets enmeshed in dark-staining red cells.
iv. The underlying atheromatous plaque may be seen.
v. Organised thrombus shows in-growth of granulation tissue at the base having spindle cells and capillary channels.

Exercise

17

Inflammation: Acute and Chronic

Objectives

- ⇨ Learn general types of inflammation with examples—acute inflammation (e.g. abscess lung, acute appendicitis), chronic inflammation (e.g. inflammatory granulation tissue).
- ⇨ Describe salient gross and microscopic features of these conditions.

ABSCESS LUNG

Abscess is formation of cavity as a result of extensive tissue necrosis following pyogenic bacterial infection accompanied by intense neutrophilic infiltration. Abscess of the lung may occur due to inhalation, embolic phenomena, and pneumonia.

G/A Abscess is more common in the right lung and may occur in upper or lower lobe. Size of the cavity may vary from small to fairly large. The wall is ragged and necrotic but advanced lesions may show fibrous and smooth wall (Fig. 17.1). The abscess may communicate with the bronchus.

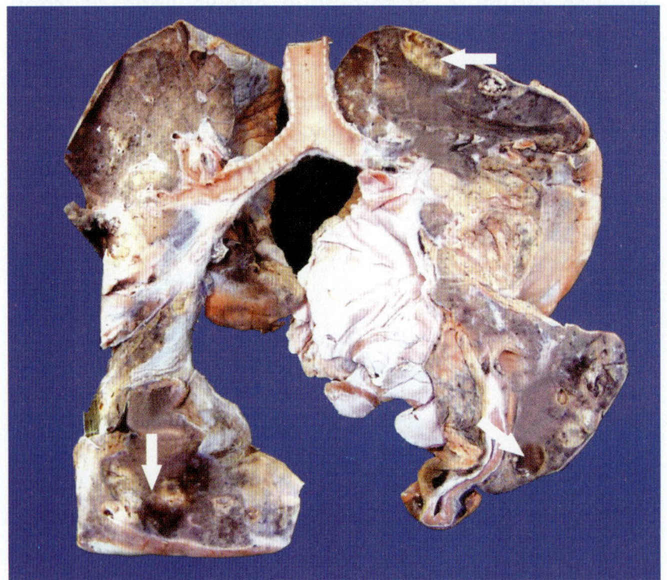

FIGURE 17.1: Lung abscess. The pleura is thickened. Cut surface of the lung shows multiple cavities 1-4 cm in diameter, having irregular and ragged inner walls (arrow). The lumina contain necrotic debris. The surrounding lung parenchyma is consolidated.

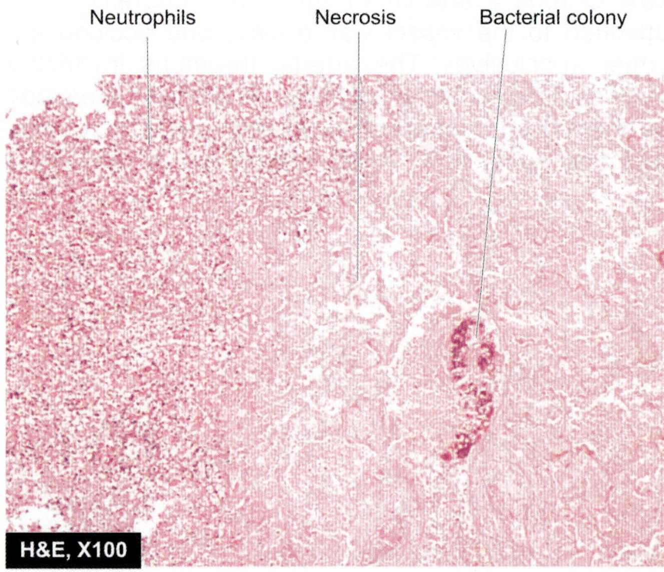

FIGURE 17.2: Lung abscess. The photomicrograph shows abscess formed by necrosed alveoli and dense acute and chronic inflammatory cells.

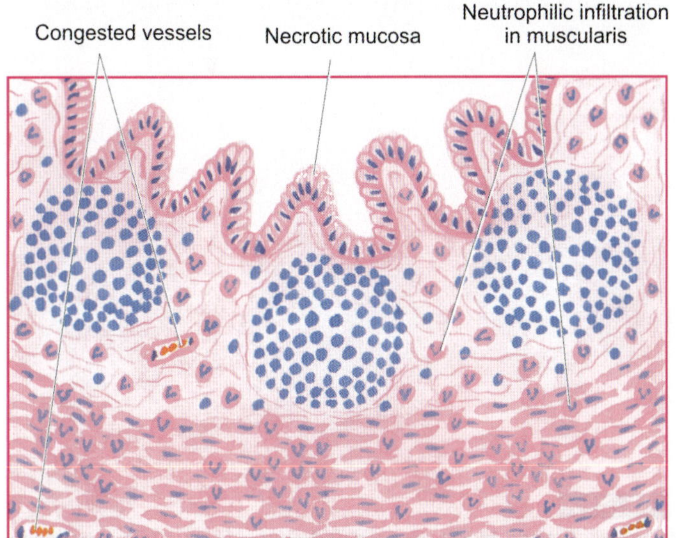

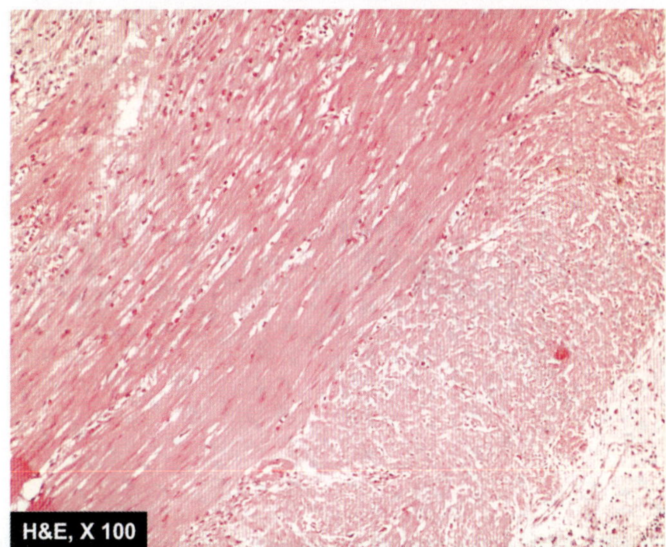

FIGURE 17.3: Acute appendicitis. Microscopic appearance showing diagnostic neutrophilic infiltration into the muscularis. Other changes present are necrosis of mucosa and periappendicitis.

M/E

i. The wall of the abscess shows dense infiltration by polymorphonuclear leucocytes and varying number of macrophages.
ii. More chronic cases show fibroblasts at the periphery.
iii. Alveolar walls in the affected area are destroyed.
iv. Lumen of the abscess contains pus consisting of purulent exudate, some red cells, fragments of tissue debris and fibrin (Fig. 17.2).

ACUTE APPENDICITIS

Acute appendicitis is the most common acute abdominal condition confronted by the surgeon.

G/A The appendix is swollen and serosa is hyperaemic and coated with fibrinopurulent exudate. The mucosa is ulcerated and sloughed.

M/E

i. Most important diagnostic feature is neutrophilic infiltration of the muscularis larger.
ii. Mucosa is sloughed and blood vessels in the wall are thrombosed.
iii. Periappendiceal inflammation is seen in advanced cases (Fig. 17.3).

CHRONIC INFLAMMATORY GRANULATION TISSUE

Granulation tissue is the granular and pink appearance of the tissue in a healing ulcer and in secondary union of wounds.

G/A Floor of the lesion contains pink granulations composed of the vascular connective tissue, while the edges are sloping and bluish-white.

M/E

i. Surface of the ulcer contains mixture of blood, fibrin and inflammatory exudate.
ii. The zone underneath contains granulation tissue composed of proliferating fibroblasts, newly-formed small blood vessels and varying number of inflammatory cells which are initially polymorphs but in the later stages macrophages and lymphocytes predominate.
iii. The epithelium grows from the edge of the wound as spurs.
iv. Granulation tissue matures from below upwards and late stage shows dense collagen, scanty vascularity and fewer inflammatory cells (Fig. 17.4).

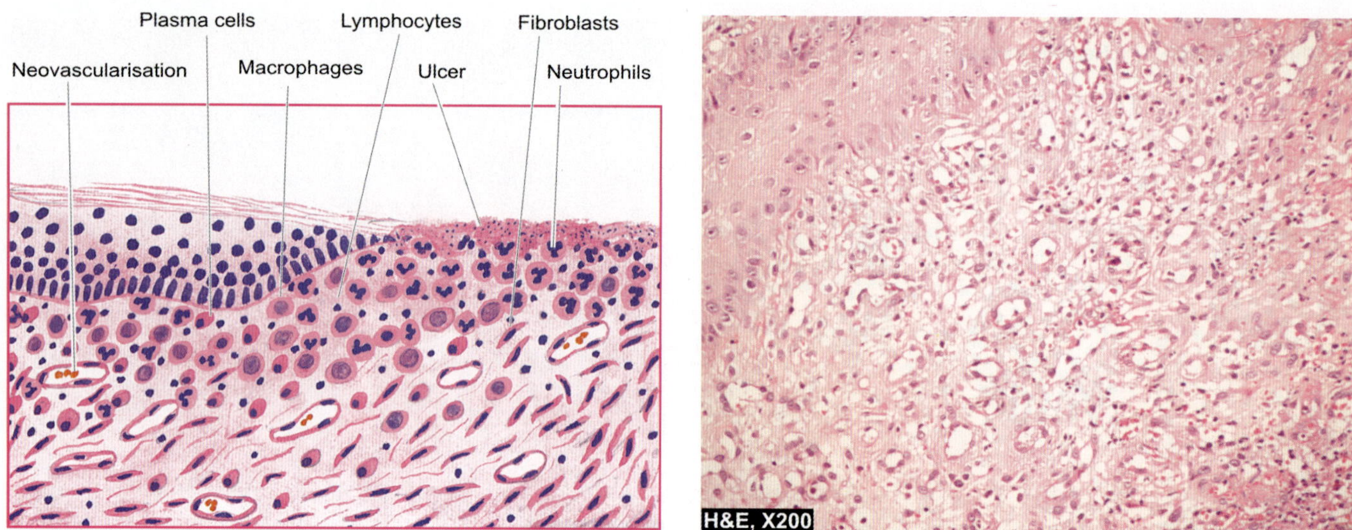

FIGURE 17.4: Active granulation tissue has inflammatory cell infiltrate, newly formed blood vessels and young fibrous tissue in loose matrix.

Exercise 18

Inflammation: Granulomatous

Objectives

- ➪ Learn granulomatous inflammation with examples—tuberculous lymphadenitis, fibrocaseous tuberculosis lung, tuberculosis intestine, military tuberculosis spleen.
- ➪ Describe salient gross and microscopic features of these conditions.

TUBERCULOUS LYMPHADENITIS

Tuberculosis of the lymph nodes is always secondary to tuberculosis elsewhere.

G/A The lymph nodes are enlarged and are matted together due to periadenitis. The cut surface in the tuberculous areas is yellow, cheesy, opaque and caseous while elsewhere it is grey brown (Fig. 18.1).

M/E

i. The caseous areas show debris composed of fragmented coagulated cells.

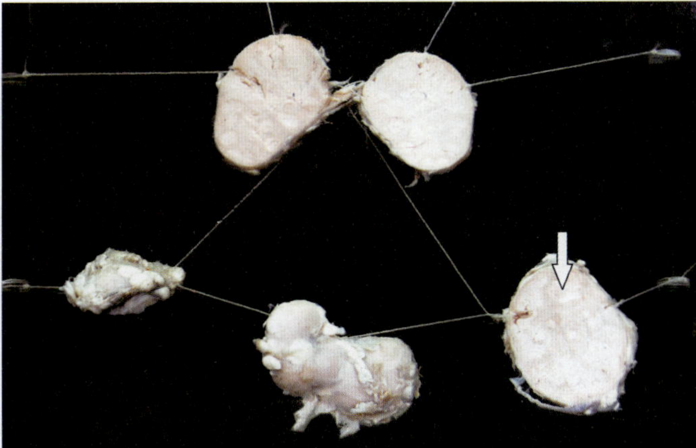

FIGURE 18.1: Tuberculous lymphadenitis. Multiple lymph nodes are matted together and surrounded by fat. Sectioned surface shows merging capsules of adjacent nodes and large areas of yellowish caseation necrosis.

ii. The periphery of caseous foci shows granulomatous inflammation consisting of epithelioid cells (identified by large size, slipper-shaped appearance, abundant pale cytoplasm and oval vesicular nuclei), surrounded by lymphocytes and some plasma cells. Epithelioid cells may fuse to form giant cells in the granuloma and may have nuclear arrangement at

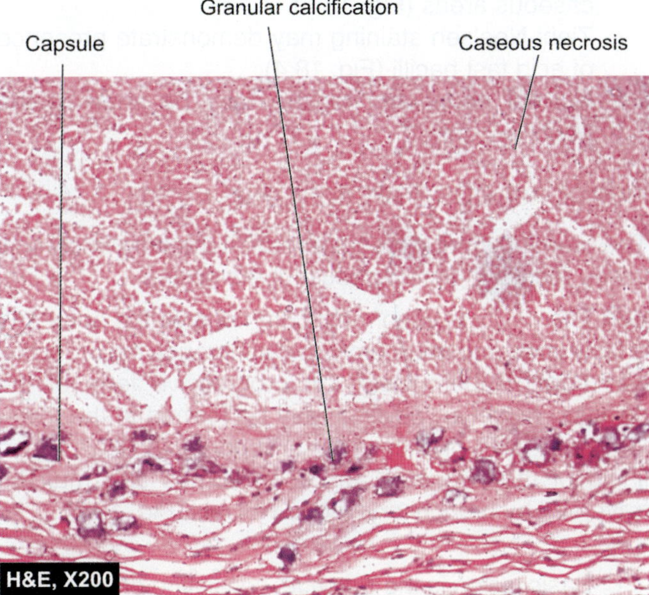

FIGURE 18.2: Tuberculous lymphadenitis. Large areas of caseation necrosis with dystrophic calcification, surrounded by epithelioid cells.

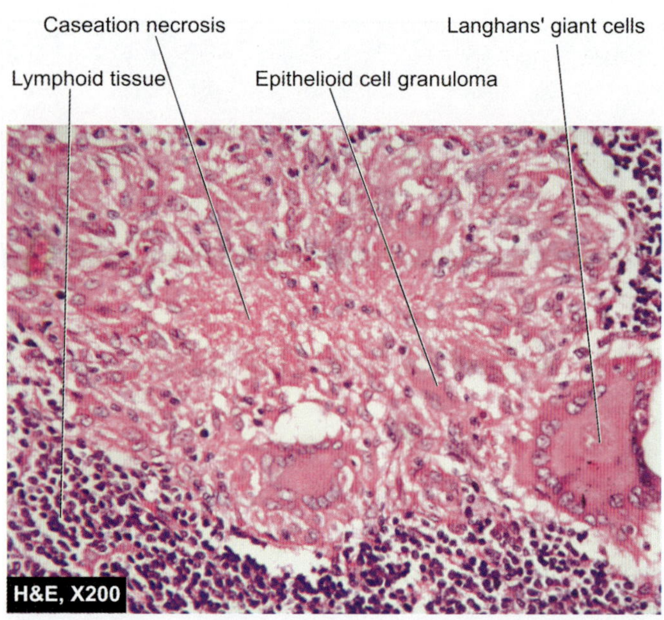

FIGURE 18.3: Tuberculous lymphadenitis. Characteristic sliper-shaped epithelioid cells, minute caseation necrosis and a Langhans' giant cell.

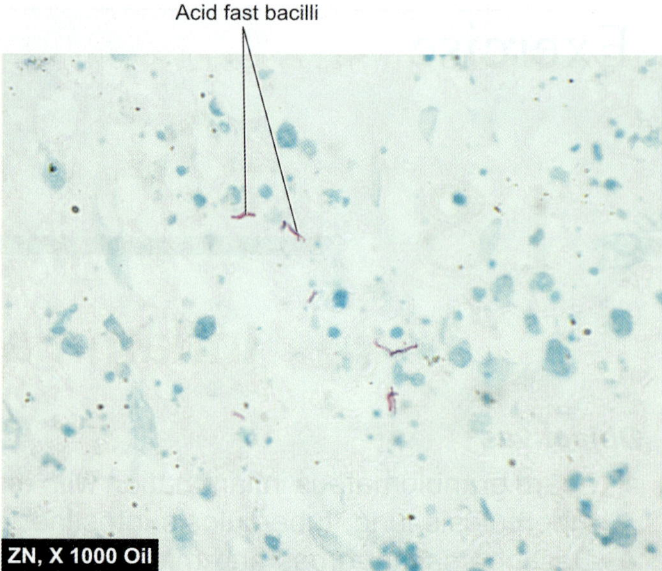

FIGURE 18.4: Tuberculous lymphadenitis. Ziehl-Neelsen staining shows the presence of acid fast bacilli.

the periphery of the cell (Langhans' giant cells) or the nuclei may be distributed haphazardly (foreign body giant cells) (Fig. 18.2).

iii. Depending upon the age of granuloma, fibroblasts may surround the granulomas.
iv. It is not uncommon to find areas of dystrophic calcification appearing as bluish granularity in the caseous areas (Fig. 18.3).
v. Ziehl-Neelsen staining may demonstrate presence of acid fast bacilli (Fig. 18.4)
v. Normal nodal architecture may be seen at the periphery only.

FIBROCASEOUS TUBERCULOSIS LUNG

The breakdown of caseous tissue in the lung in chronic cases results in fibrocaseous tuberculosis.

G/A The cavity is seen most commonly at the apex and is fairly large and may communicate through the bronchial wall ('open tuberculosis'). In progressive form of the disease, however, cavities may be formed in the lower lobe too. Wall of the cavity is smooth (unlike ragged lining of the pyogenic abscess), fibrous and may be traversed by bronchi and blood vessels (Fig. 18.5).

M/E

i. Basic lesion is the *tubercle*, consisting of epithelioid cells, lymphocytes and giant cells, and central area of caseation necrosis. The tubercles coalesce to form confluent areas.
ii. Periphery of the lesion shows proliferating fibroblasts and fibrosis (Fig. 18.6).
iii. The arteries may show endarteritis obliterans closing the lumen.
iv. The surrounding alveoli may contain cellular exudate.

TUBERCULOSIS INTESTINE

Intestinal tuberculosis occurs in 3 forms: primary, secondary and hyperplastic. Secondary tuberculosis of the small intestine is most common.

G/A The intestine shows large ulcers which are transverse to the long axis of the bowel. These ulcers may be

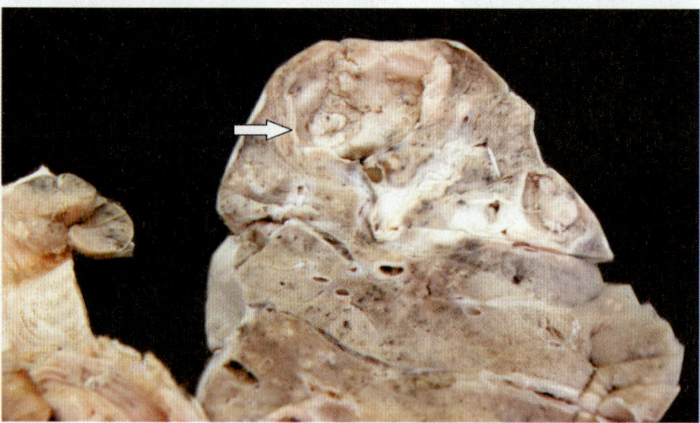

FIGURE 18.5: Chronic fibrocaseous tuberculosis lung. Sectioned surface of the lung shows a cavity in the apex of the lung (arrow). The cavity is lined by yellowish caseous necrotic material. The lung tissue around the cavity is consolidated.

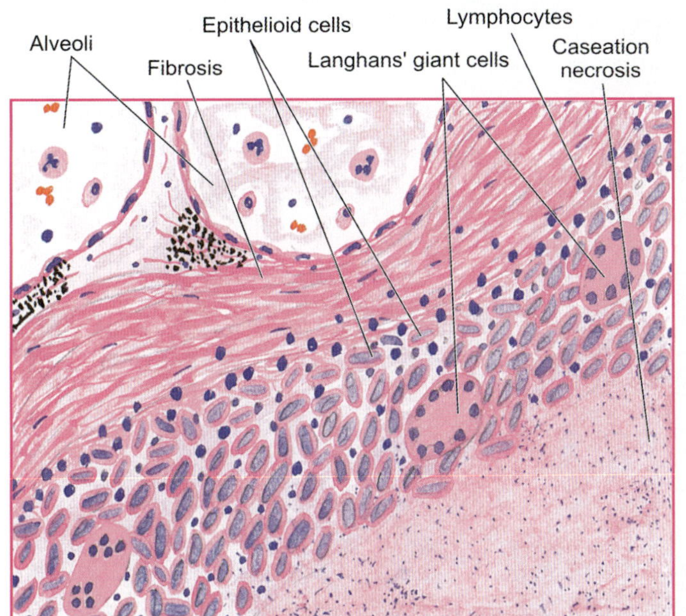

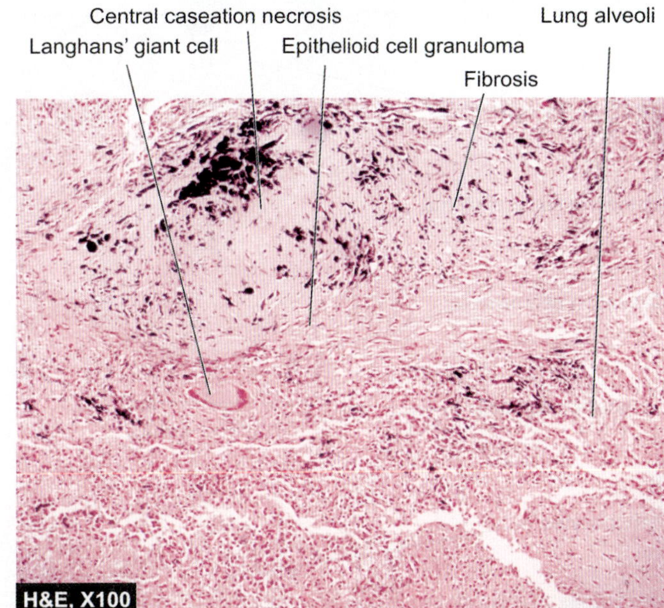

FIGURE 18.6: Fibrocaseous tuberculosis lung. The cavity shows caseation necrosis while the wall shows epithelioid cells admixed with lymphocytes and some Langhans' giant cells and surrounded at the periphery by fibrosclerosis.

coated with caseous material. Advanced cases show transverse fibrous strictures and intestinal obstruction (Fig. 18.7).

M/E

i. Presence of caseating tubercles in all the layers of intestine (Fig. 18.8).
ii. Ulceration of mucosa with slough on the surface.
iii. Variable fibrosis in the muscular layer.

MILIARY TUBERCULOSIS SPLEEN

Lymphohaematogenous spread of chronic pulmonary tuberculosis may result in acute miliary tuberculosis of the spleen.

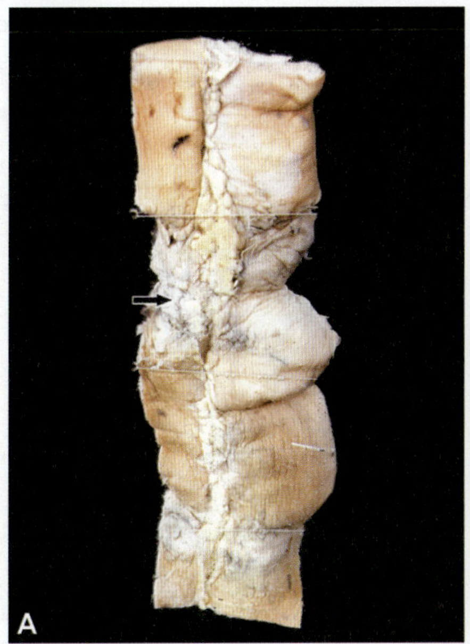

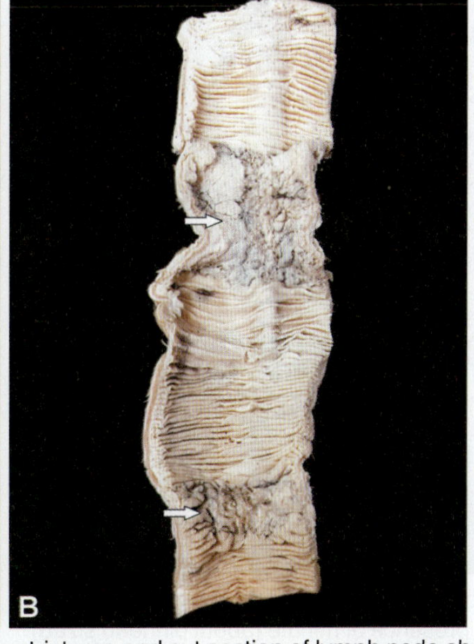

FIGURE 18.7: Intestinal tuberculosis. A, The external surface shows strictures and cut section of lymph node showing caseation necrosis (black arrow). B, The lumen shows transverse ulcers and strictures (transverse to the long axis of intestine) (arrows). The intestinal wall has multiple transverse strictures where the intestinal wall is thickened and grey-white and mucosa over it is ulcerated.

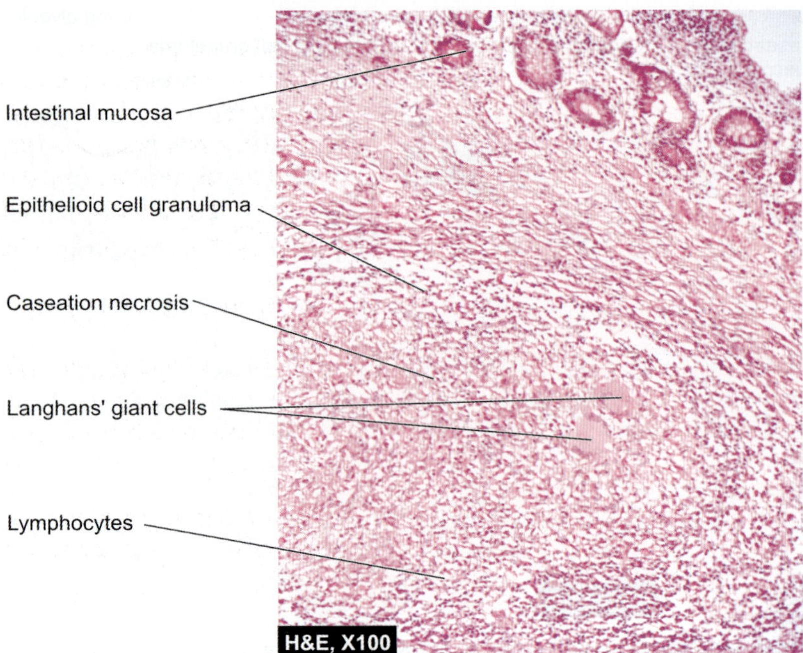

FIGURE 18.8: Tuberculosis small intestine. The wall of intestine shows caseating epithelioid cell granulomas.

G/A The miliary tubercles are scattered throughout the liver. They appear as yellowish-white firm lesions of a few millimeter in diameter (Fig. 18.9).

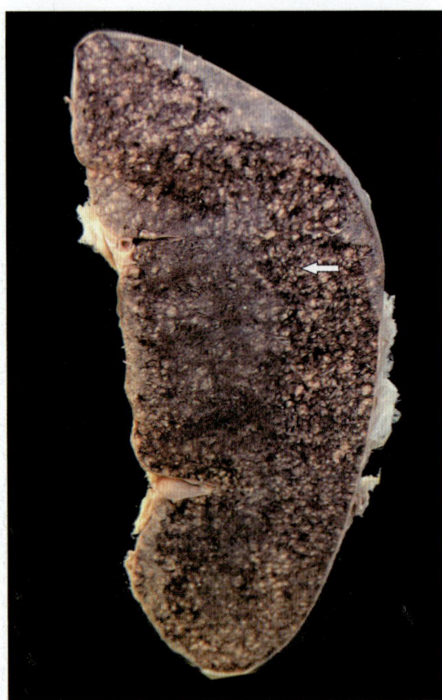

FIGURE 18.9: Miliary tuberculosis spleen. The capsule as well as sectioned surface shows presence of minute (about pinhead sized) yellowish nodules with central necrosis called tubercles (arrow).

M/E

i. Tubercles with minute areas of central caseation necrosis are seen scattered in the splenic parenchyma.
ii. The neighbouring splenic parenchyma may show congestion (Fig. 18.10).

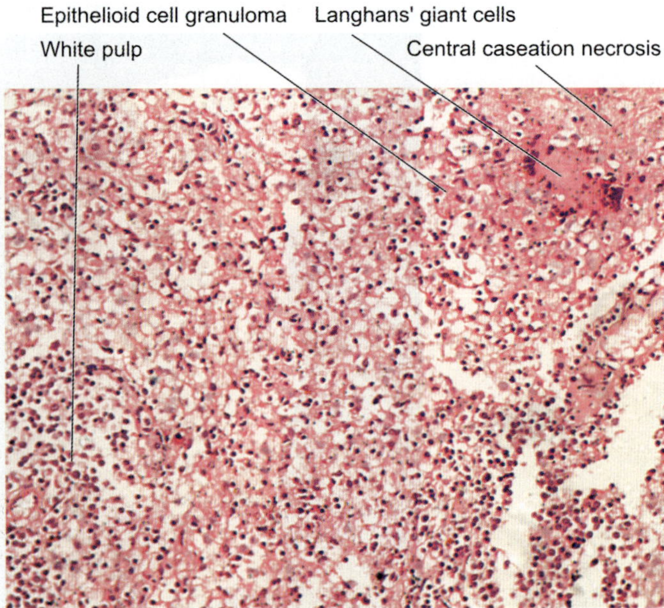

FIGURE 18.10: Miliary tuberculosis spleen. Small caseating granuloma is seen in the splenic tissue.

Exercise

19

Other Specific Infections and Infestations

Objectives

- ⇨ Learn common examples of other bacterial (e.g. actinomycosis skin), fungal (e.g. aspergillosis lung, rhinosporidiosis nose) and parasitic (e.g. cysticercosis soft tissue) infections.
- ⇨ Describe salient gross and microscopic features of these conditions.

ACTINOMYCOSIS SKIN

Actinomycosis is a chronic suppurative disease caused by anaerobic bacteria, *Actinomyces israelii.* Head and neck region is the most common location of the lesion.

G/A There is a firm swelling in the region of the lower jaw initially but later sinuses and abscesses are formed. The pus contains characteristic yellow *sulphur granules* (Fig. 19.1).

M/E

i. The inflammatory reaction is a granuloma with central suppuration. Centre of the lesion shows abscess and at the periphery are seen chronic inflammatory cells, giant cells and fibroblasts.
ii. The bacterial colony, sulphur granule, is characterised by basophilic radiating filaments, hence also termed 'ray fungus'.
iii. The periphery of the granule has hyaline, eosinophilic, club-like ends best highlighted by Masson's trichrome stain (Fig. 19.2).

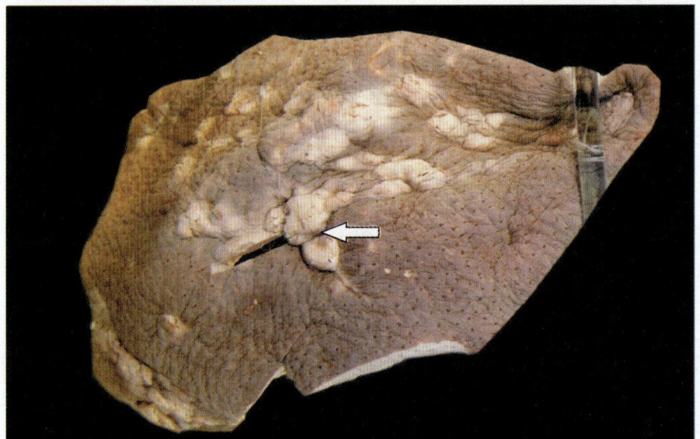

FIGURE 19.1: Skin surface shows multiple draining sinuses with blackish grains (arrow). These sinuses extend into underlying tissues as well.

ASPERGILLOSIS LUNG

Aspergillosis is the most common opportunistic fungal infection, usually involving the lungs. The most common human pathogen is *Aspergillus fumigatus*. It occurs in 3 forms—allergic bronchopulmonary aspergillosis, aspergilloma and invasive aspergillosis.

G/A Aspergillosis occurs in pulmonary cavities or in bronchiectasis as fungal ball.

M/E

i. There is a mass of tangled hyphae lying within a cavity with fibrous wall.
ii. The organism has characteristic septate hyphae (2-7 μm in diameter) and has multiple diochotomous branching at acute angles (Fig. 19.3). These can be highlighted by special stain, Gomori's methenamine silver (GMS) or periodic acid Schiff (PAS) (Fig. 19.4).
iii. The wall of cavity shows chronic inflammatory cells.

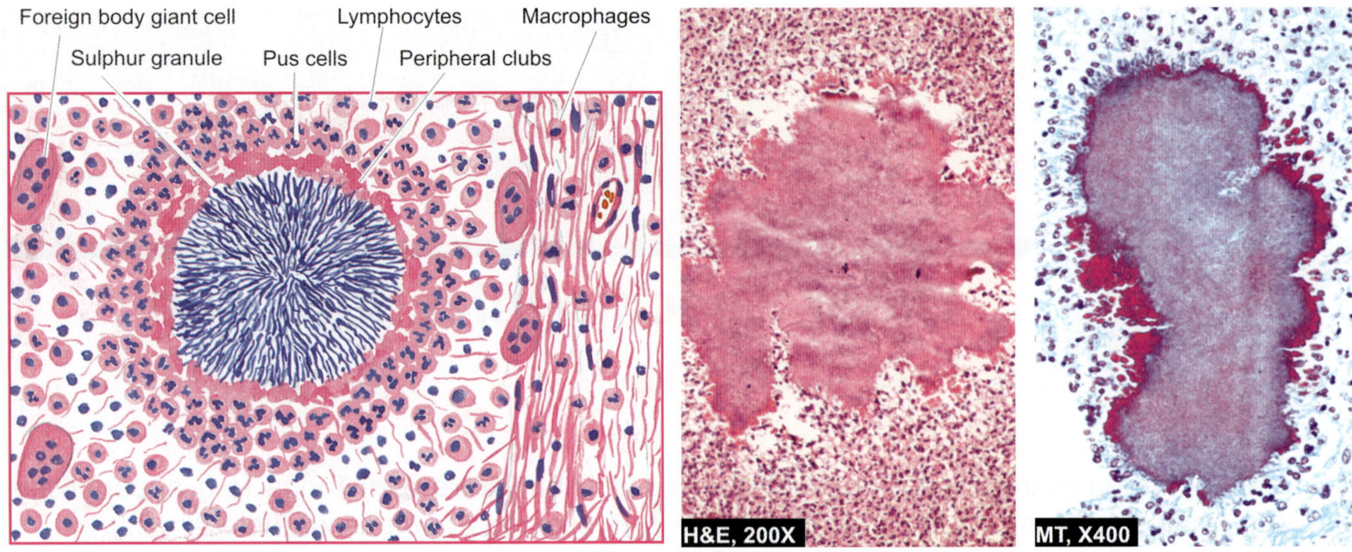

FIGURE 19.2: Actinomycosis. Microscopic appearance of sulphur granule lying inside an abscess. The margin of the colony shows hyaline filaments highlighted by Masson's trichrome stain (right photomicrograph).

RHINOSPORIDIOSIS NOSE

Rhinosporidiosis of the nose is caused by the fungus, *Rhinosporidium seeberi.*

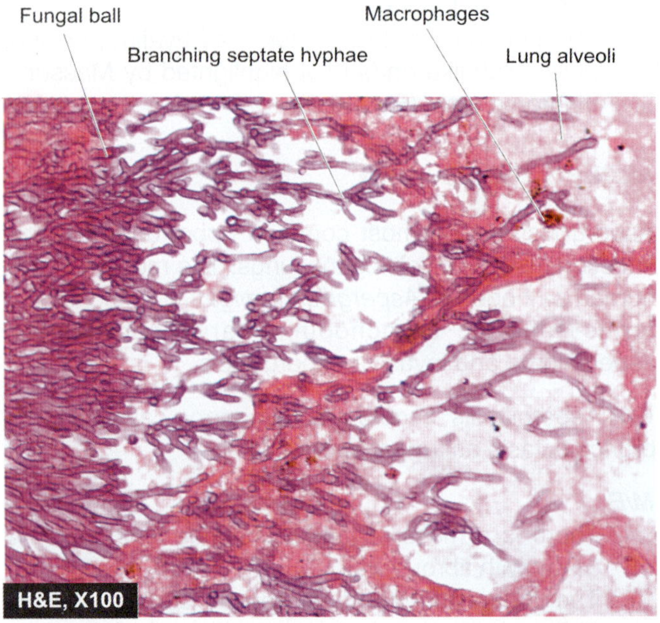

FIGURE 19.3: Aspergillosis lung. Acute angled septate hyphae lying in necrotic debris and acute inflammatory exudates in lung abscess.

G/A Rhinosporidiosis occurs in a nasal polyp typically. The polypoid mass is gelatinous with smooth and shining surface.

M/E

i. Structure of nasal polyp of inflammatory or allergic type is seen i.e. subepithelial loose oedematous connective tissue containing mucous glands and varying number of inflammatory cells like lymphocytes, plasma cells and eosinophils. The surface of the polyp is covered by respiratory epithelium which may show squamous metaplasia.
ii. Large number of organisms of the size of erythrocytes with chitinous wall are seen in the thick-walled sporangia. Spores are also seen in the submucosa and on the surface of the mucosa (Fig. 19.5).

CYSTICERCOSIS SOFT TISSUE

Cysticercus cellulosae is caused by the larval stage of pork tapeworm, *Taenia solium.* The most common sites in the body are skeletal muscle, brain, skin and heart.

G/A The lesions may be solitary or multiple and appear as round to oval white cyst, about 1 cm in diameter (Fig. 19.6). The cyst contains milky fluid.

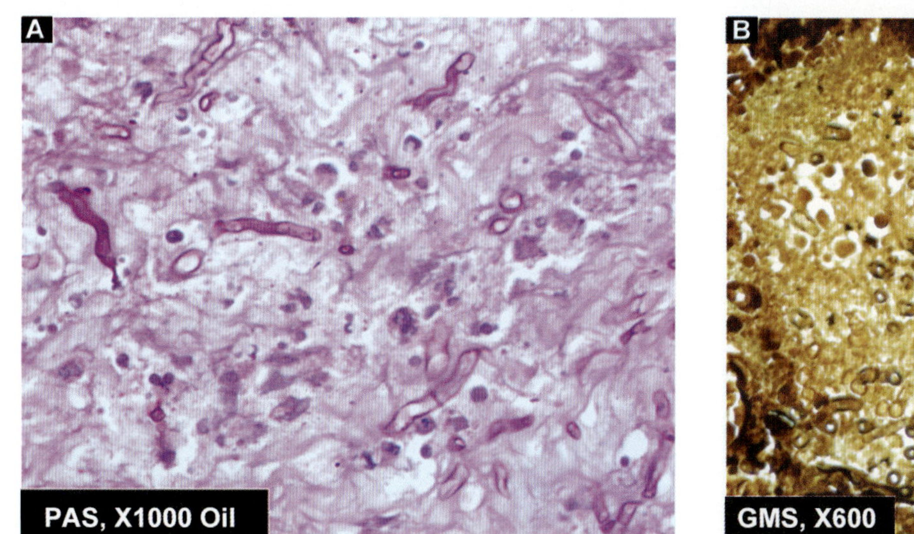

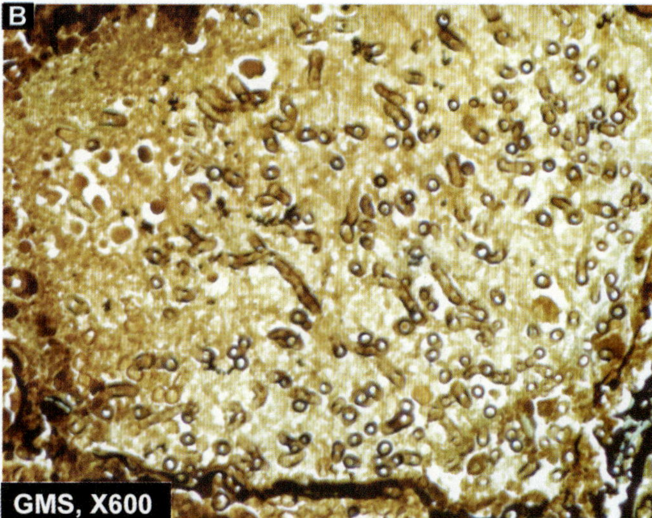

FIGURE 19.4: Aspergillosis lung. Organisms, *Apergillus flavus*, are best identified with a special stain for fungi, Periodic acid Schiff (PAS) stain (A) and Gomori's methenamine silver (GMS) (B).

M/E

i. The cysticercus cellulosae lying in the cyst shows continuity of epithelium on surface and that lining the body canal. Sometimes the parasite is degenerated or even calcified.
ii. The dead and degenerated forms incite intense tissue reaction. This reaction is in the form of palisades of histiocytes, surrounded by inflammatory cell reaction consisting of mixed infiltrate including prominence of eosinophils (Fig. 19.7).

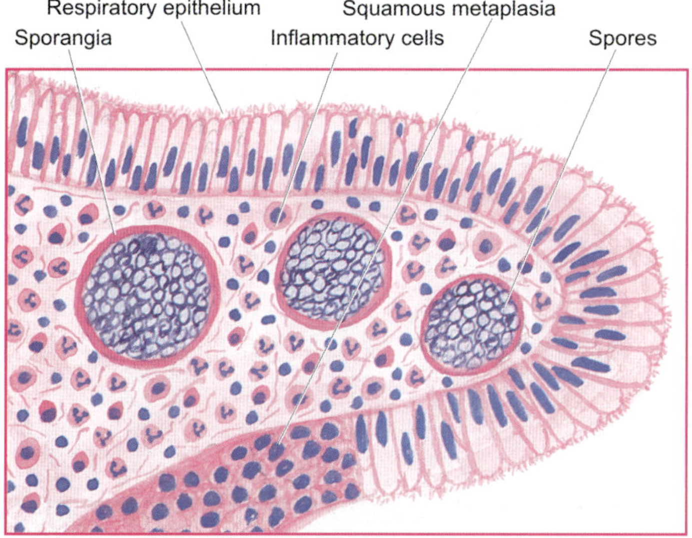

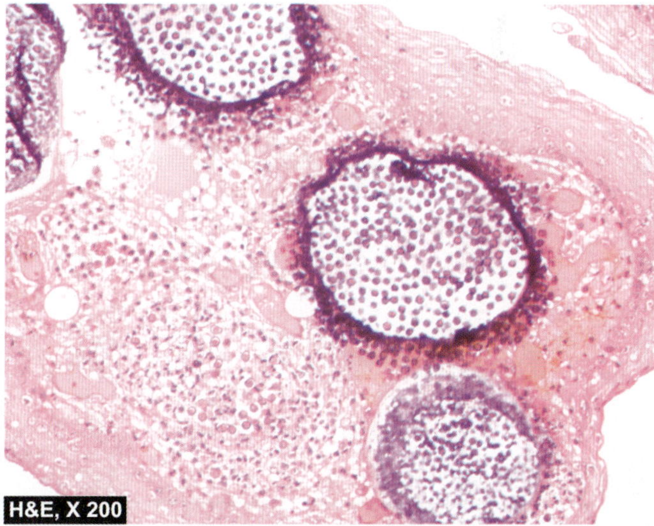

FIGURE 19.5: Rhinosporidiosis in a nasal polyp. The spores are present in sporangia as well as are intermingled in the inflammatory cell infiltrate.

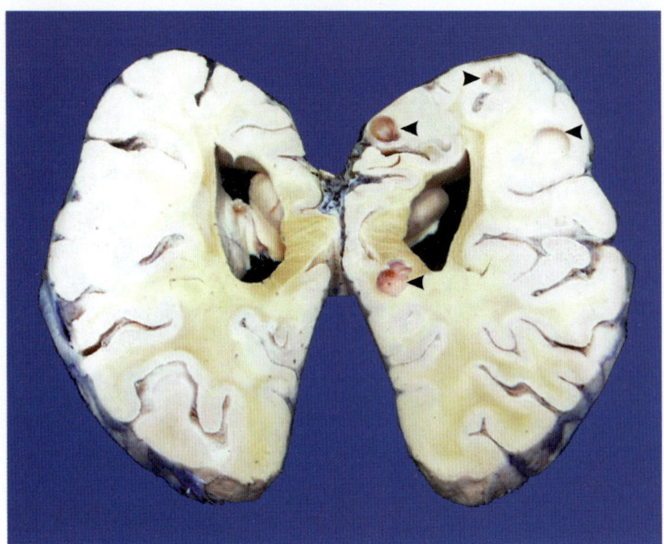

FIGURE 19.6: Neurocysticercosis. The sliced surface of the cerebral hemisphere of the brain shows many tiny whitish nodules and cysts about 1 cm in diameter.

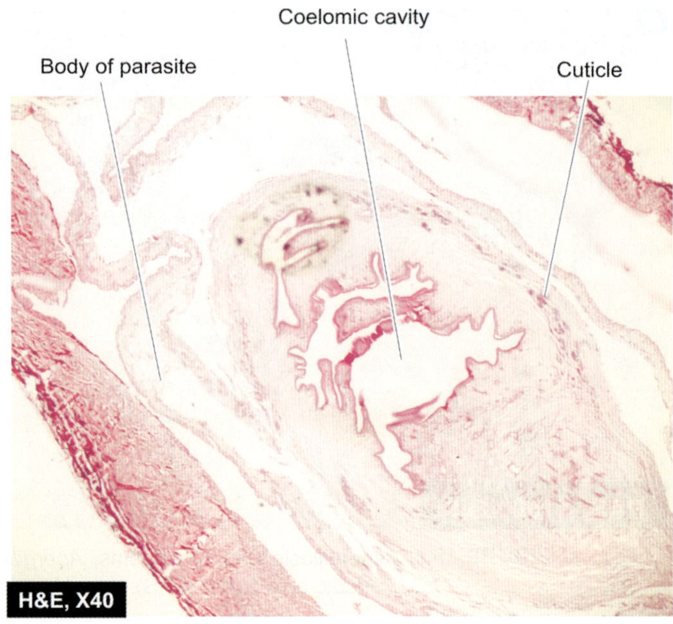

FIGURE 19.7: Cysticercus cellulosae. The worm is seen in the cyst while the cyst wall shows palisade layer of histiocytes.

Exercise

20 Common Primary Epithelial Tumours—I

Objectives

- ⇨ Learn common examples of primary benign and malignant epithelial tumours of the skin and mucosa (e.g. squamous cell papilloma, squamous cell carcinoma, adenoma, adenocarcinoma).
- ⇨ Describe salient gross and microscopic features of these conditions.

SQUAMOUS CELL PAPILLOMA

Squamous cell papilloma is a common benign epithelial tumour of the skin.

G/A Surface of the tumour shows finger-like processes (Fig. 20.1).

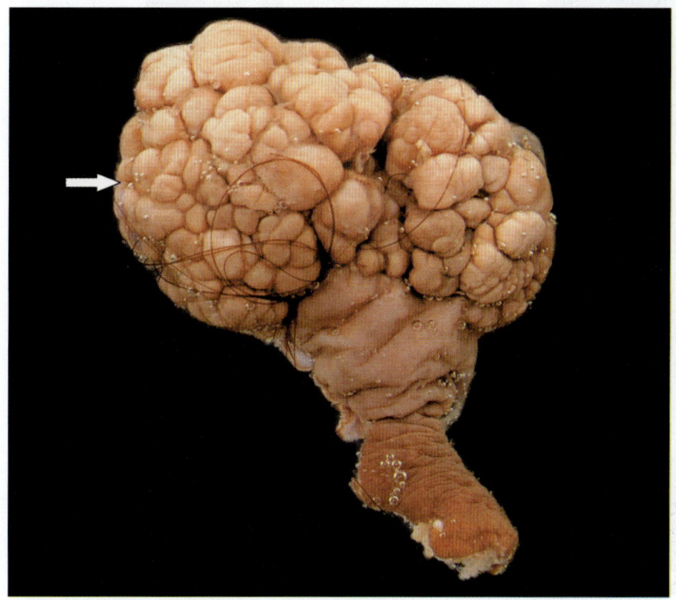

FIGURE 20.1: Squamous cell papilloma skin. The skin surface shows a papillary growth on the surface (arrow) having a pedicle. It is elevated above the adjoining normal skin without any invasion.

M/E

i. The epidermis is thickened but orderly and is thrown into finger-like processes or papillae.
ii. The central core of the papillae is composed of loose fibrovascular tissue (Fig. 20.2).

SQUAMOUS CELL CARCINOMA

Squamous cell or epidermoid carcinoma occurs most commonly in the skin, oral cavity, oesophagus, uterine cervix, penis, lungs and at the edge of chronic ulcers.

G/A The tumour is either in the form of nodular and ulcerative growth, or fungating and polypoid mass without ulceration. The margin of the growth is elevated and indurated. Cut section of the growth shows grey-white endophytic as well as exophytic tumour (Fig. 20.3).

M/E

i. The tumour is characterised by malignant cells which may show variable degree of differentiation.
ii. The masses of tumour cells invade through the basement membrane into dermis.
iii. In better differentiated tumours, the cells are arranged in concentric layers called epithelial pearls and contain keratin material in the centre of the cell masses.
iv. The masses of tumour cells are separated by lymphocytes (Figs 20.4).

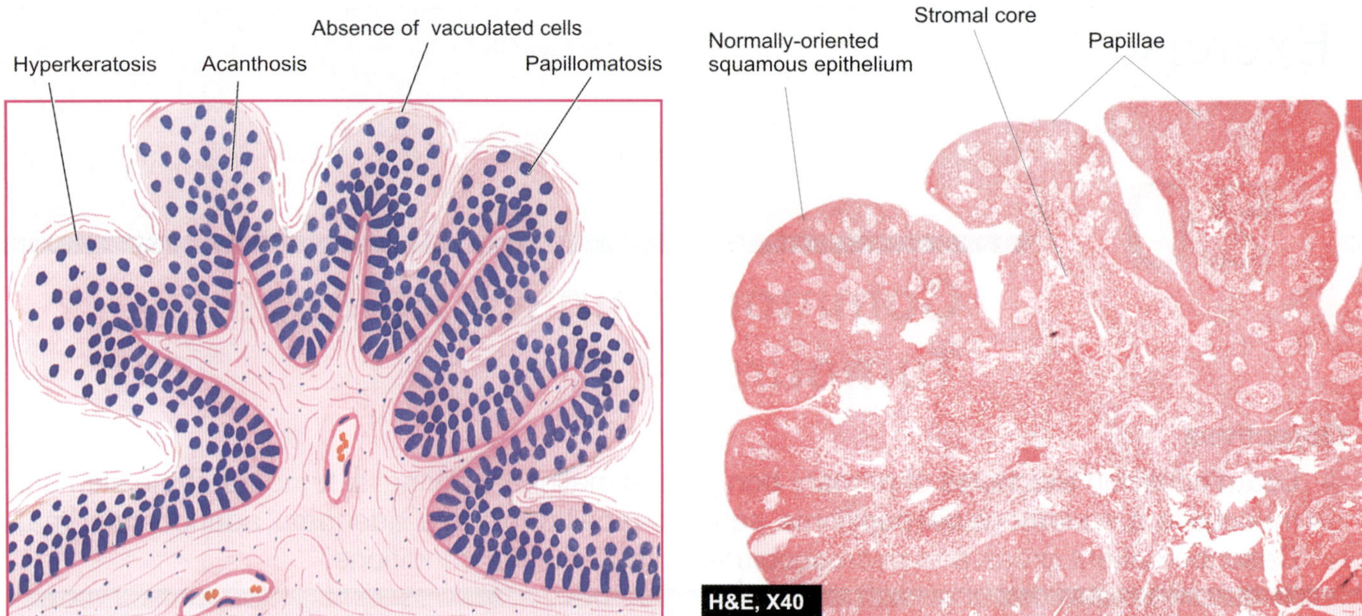

FIGURE 20.2: Papilloma skin. Finger-like projections are covered by normally-oriented squamous epithelium while the stromal core contains fibrovascular tissue.

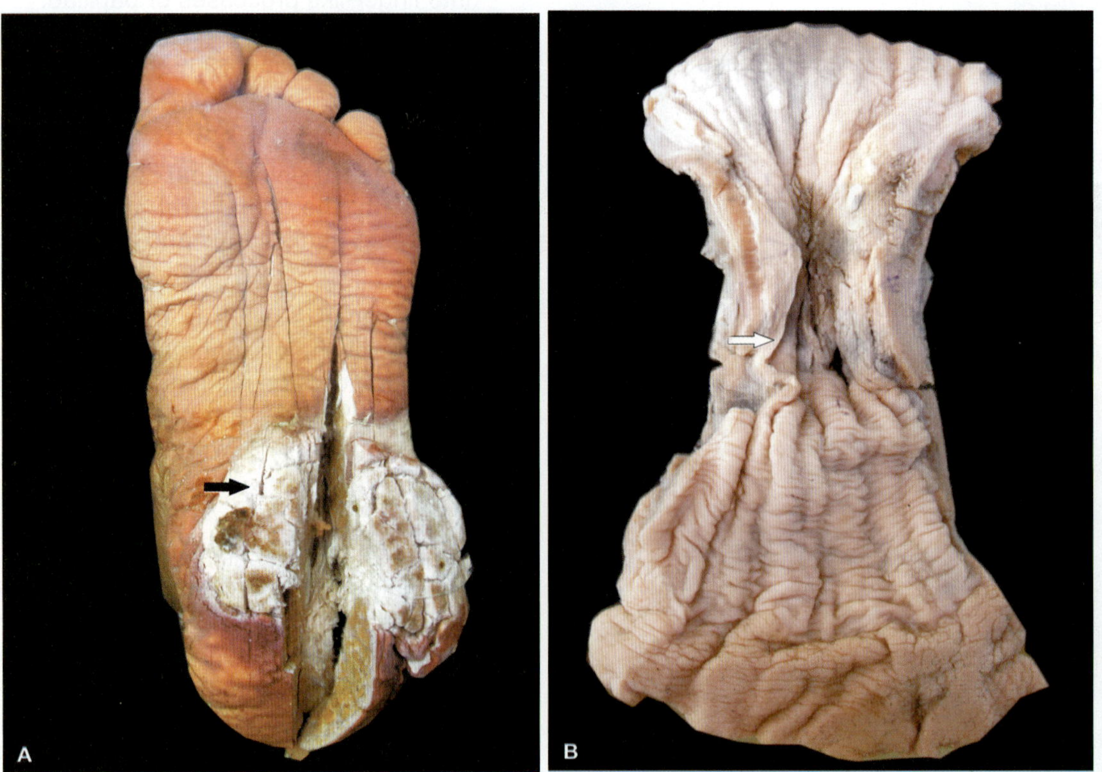

FIGURE 20.3: Squamous cell carcinoma. A, The skin surface on the sole of the foot shows a fungating and ulcerated growth (arrow). B, Carcinoma oesophagus showing narrowing of the lumen and thickening of the wall (arrow).

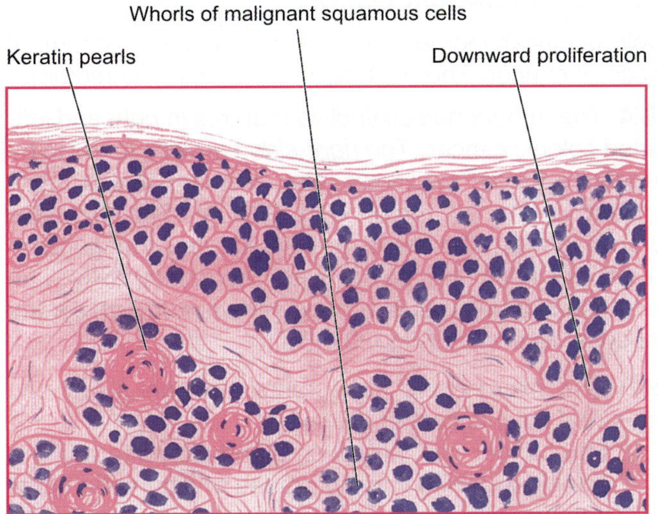

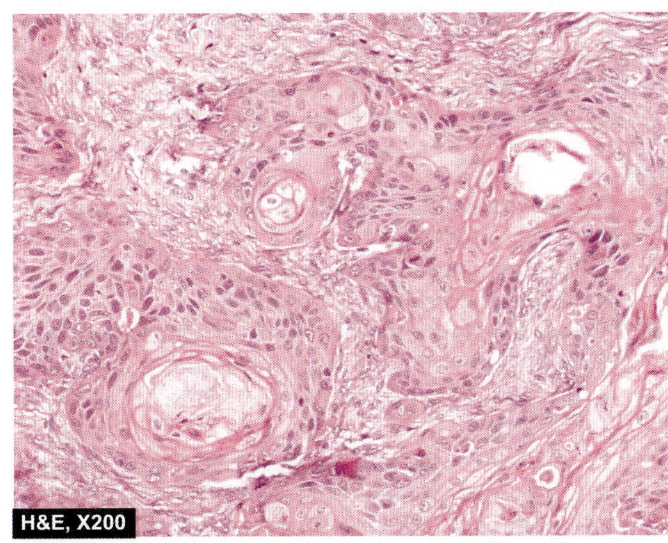

FIGURE 20.4: Squamous cell carcinoma, well-differentiated type. The dermis is invaded by downward proliferating epidermal masses of cells which show atypical features. A few horn pearls with central laminated keratin are present. There is marked inflammatory reaction in the dermis between the masses of tumour cells.

ADENOMA RECTUM

Colorectal adenomas are neoplastic (adenomatous) polyps which have potential for malignant change.

Adenomas have 3 main varieties (tubular, villous and tubulovillous), each of which represents a difference in the growth pattern of the same neoplastic process and variable biological behaviour.

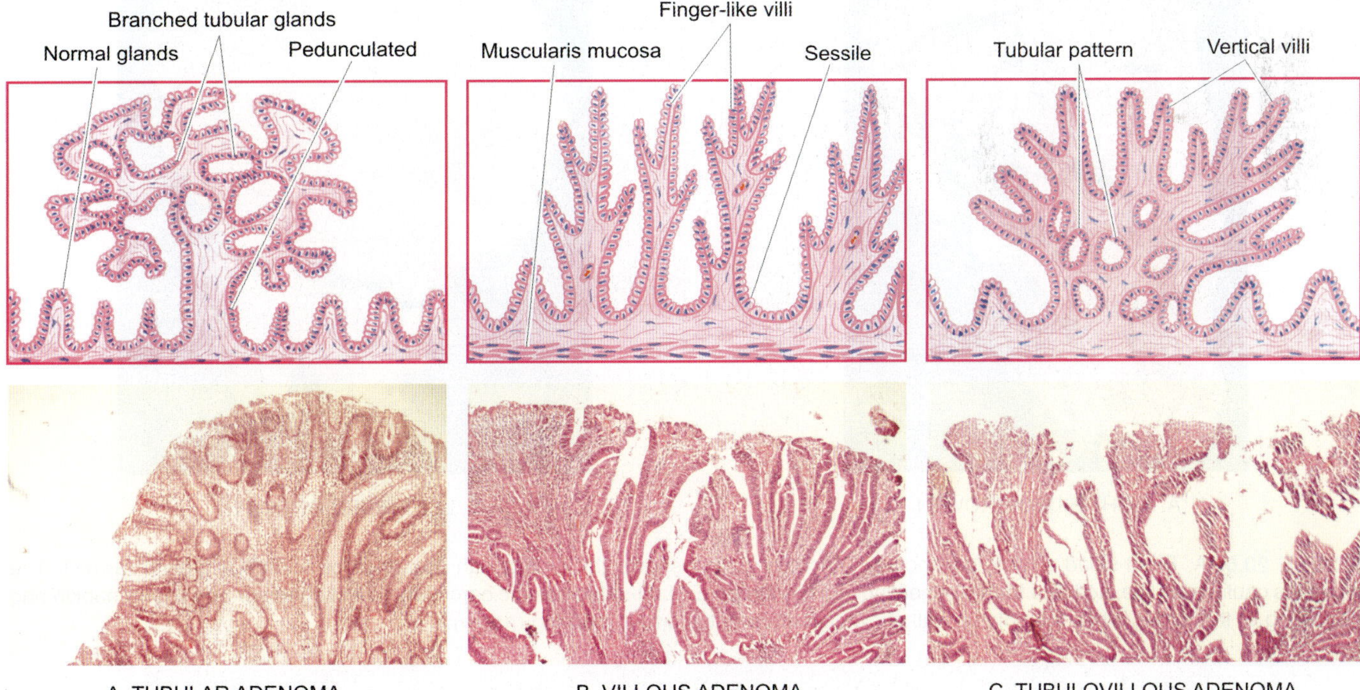

FIGURE 20.5: Colorectal adenoma—tubular type (adenomatous polyp). The polypoid lesion is covered by mucosa having flat surface. The stroma contains many tubule-like formations of gland showing variable atypia.

G/A The adenomatous polyps may be single or multiple, sessile or pedunculated, vary in size from less than 1 cm to large, spherical masses with an irregular surface. Usually, the larger lesions have recognisable stalks.

M/E

i. Tubular adenoma is a benign tumour overlying the muscularis mucosa.
ii. It is composed of branching tubules which are embedded in the lamina propria.
iii. The lining epithelial cells are of large intestinal type with diminished mucus secreting capacity, large nuclei and increased mitotic activity (Fig. 20.5).
iv. It may show variable degree of cytologic atypia ranging from atypical epithelium restricted within the glandular basement membrane called as 'carcinoma *in situ*' to invasion into the fibrovascular stromal core termed as frank adenocarcinoma.

ADENOCARCINOMA COLON

Colorectal carcinoma comprises the commonest form of visceral cancer. The most common location is rectum.

G/A The tumour has distinctive features in right and left-sided colonic cancer. *The right-sided growth*, tends to be fungating, large, cauliflower-like, soft and friable mass projecting into the lumen (Fig. 20.6,A). The *left-sided growth*, on the other hand, has napkin-ring configuration i.e. it encircles the bowel wall circumferentially with increased fibrous tissue forming annular ring with central mucosal ulceration (Fig. 20.6,B).

M/E The microscopic appearance on right-sided and left-sided colonic cancer is similar:

i. The tumour has infiltrating glandular pattern in the colonic wall with varying grades of differentiation of tumour cells.
ii. About 10% cases show mucin-secreting colloid carcinoma with pools of mucin (Fig. 20.7).

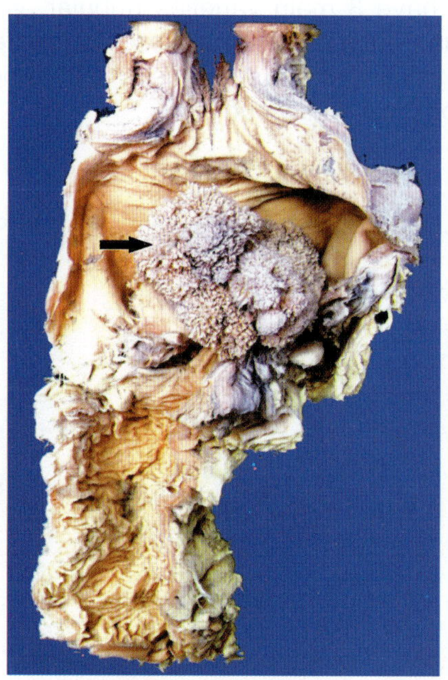

A, RIGHT-SIDED GROWTH

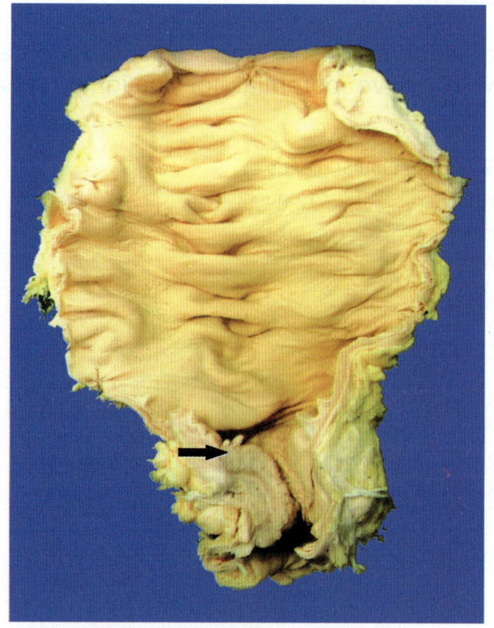

B, LEFT-SIDED GROWTH

FIGURE 20.6: A, Right-sided colonic carcinoma. The colonic wall shows thickening with presence of a luminal growth (arrow). The growth is cauliflower-like, soft and friable projecting into the lumen. B, Left-sided colonic carcinoma. Sectioned surface shows napkin ring narrowing of the lumen while the colonic wall shows circumferential firm thickening (arrow).

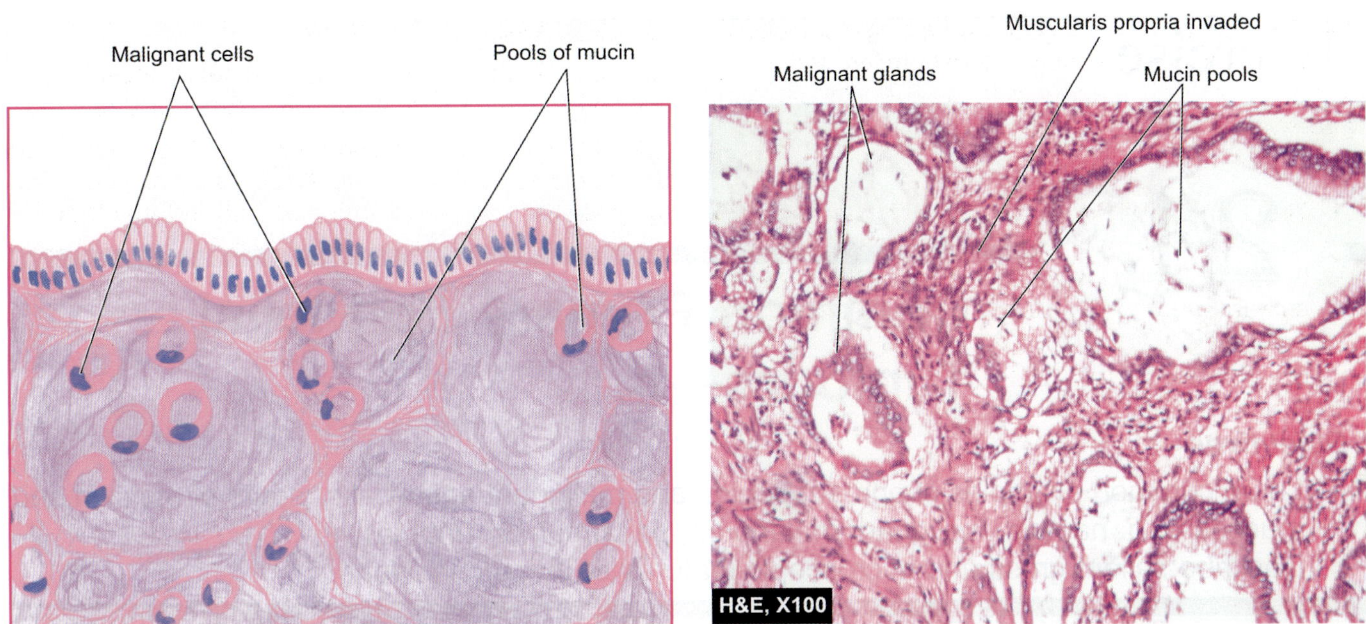

FIGURE 20.7: Mucinous adenocarcinoma colon. Pools of extracellular mucin as well as intracellular mucin in malignant glands.

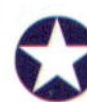

Exercise

21 Common Primary Epithelial Tumours—II

Objectives

- ⇨ Learn common examples of primary benign and malignant epithelial tumours of the skin and mucosa (e.g. naevus, malignant melanoma, basal cell carcinoma).
- ⇨ Describe salient gross and microscopic features of these conditions.

COMPOUND NAEVUS

Common moles or naevi (more appropriately termed nevocellular naevi) are the common benign neoplasms of the skin arising from melanocytes. There are numerous clinical and histologic types of nevocellular naevi and have variable clinical appearance.

G/A Grossly and clinically, a mole initially appears as a small tan dot 0.1-0.2 cm in diameter but subsequently enlarges to a uniform coloured tan to brown area which may be flat or slightly elevated and having regular, circular or oval outline.

M/E

i. The lesion is composed of melanocytes forming aggregates or nests at the dermo-epidermal junction (junctional naevus) which subsequently migrate to the underlying dermis (compound naevus). The older lesions may be entirely confined to dermis (dermal naevus).

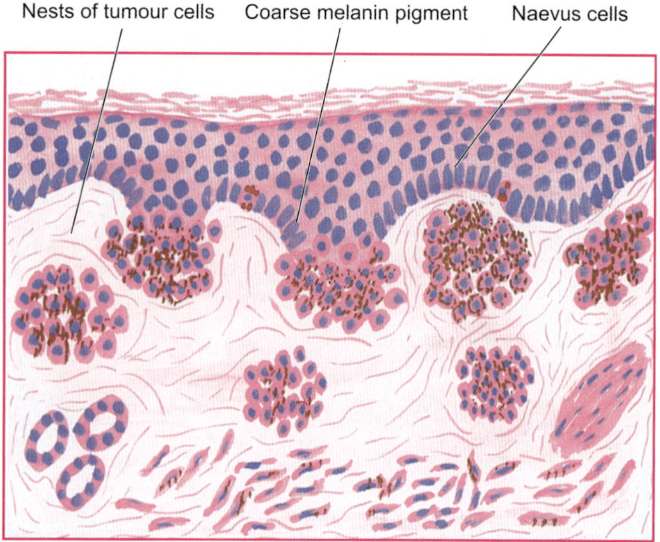

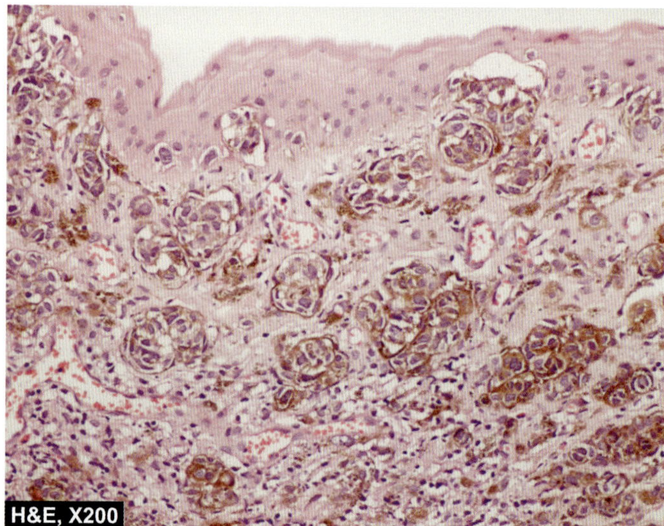

FIGURE 21.1: Compound naevus showing clusters of benign naevus cells in the dermis as well as in lower epidermis. These cells contain coarse, granular, brown-black melanin pigment.

ii. The melanocytes forming naevi are round to oval cells and have round or oval nuclei. The cytoplasm of naevus cells is homogeneous and contains abundant granular coarse brown-black melanin pigment (Fig. 21.1).
iii. The pigment is more marked in the naevus cells in the lower epidermis and upper dermis but the cells in the mid-dermis and lower dermis hardly contain any pigment.

MALIGNANT MELANOMA

Malignant melanoma or melanocarcinoma is the malignant counterpart of naevus and is the most rapidly spreading malignant tumour of the skin.

G/A Malignant melanoma may appear as flat, macular or slightly elevated, nodular lesion. The lesion exhibits variation in pigmentation appearing in shades of black, brown, grey, blue or red. The borders are irregular (Fig. 21.2).

M/E

i. The tumour has marked junctional activity at the epidermo-dermal junction and grows horizontally as well as downwards into the dermis.
ii. The tumour cells are arranged in a variety of patterns—solid masses, sheets, islands etc.

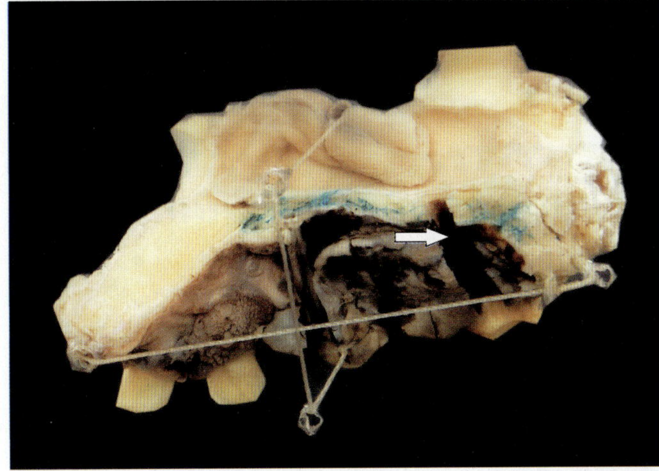

FIGURE 21.2: Malignant melanoma oral cavity. In this hemimaxillectomy specimen, whitish oral mucosa shows an elevated blackish area with ulceration. Cut surface shows blackish tumour with irregular outlines (arrow).

iii. The individual tumour cells are usually larger than the naevus cells, contain large vesicular nuclei with peripherally condensed chromatin and having prominent eosinophilic nucleoli. The cytoplasm is amphophilic (Fig. 21.3).
iv. Melanin pigment is present in the cytoplasm in the form of uniform fine granules (unlike coarse pigment granules in cells at the periphery of the lesion).

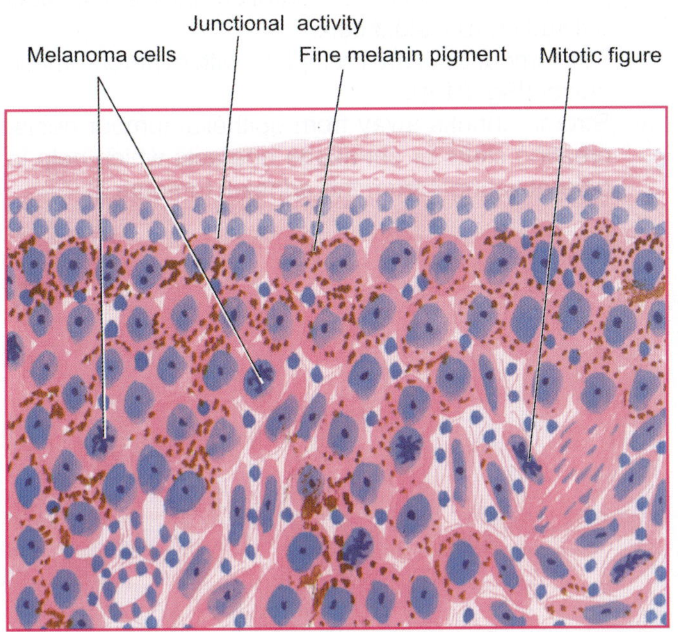

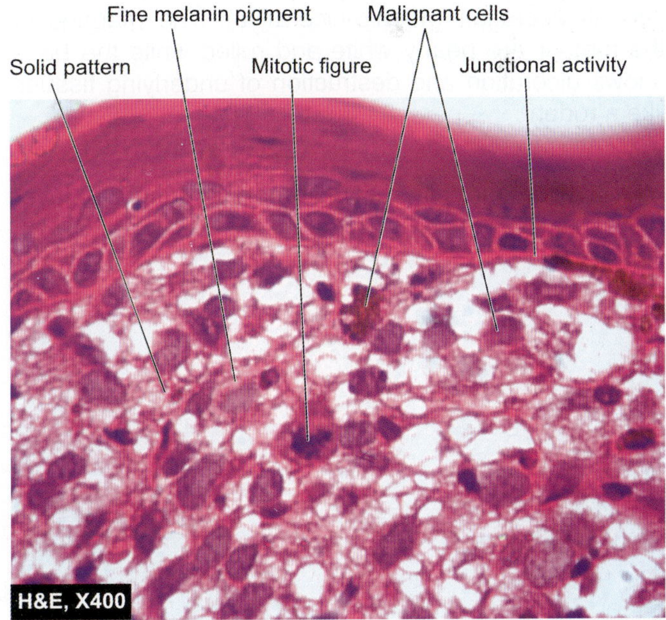

FIGURE 21.3: Malignant melanoma. There is marked junctional activity at the dermal-epidermal junction. Tumour cells resembling epithelioid cells with pleomorphic nuclei and prominent nucleoli are seen as solid masses in the dermis. Many of the tumour cells contain fine granular melanin pigment.

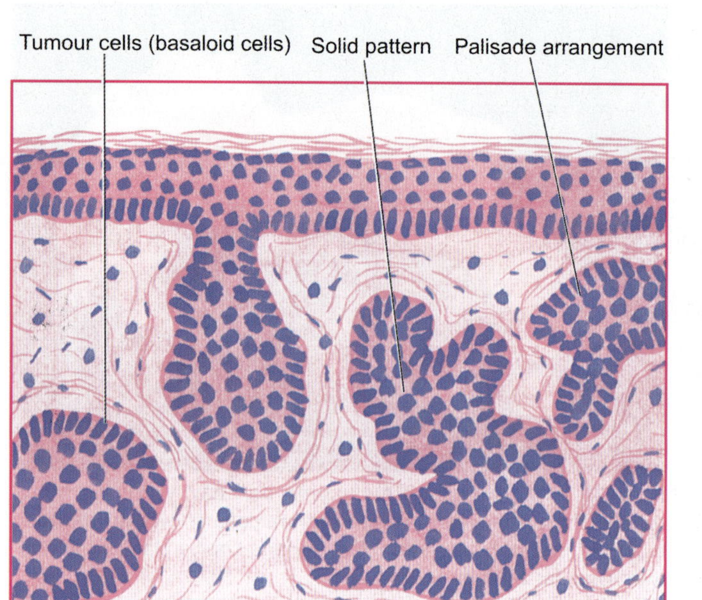

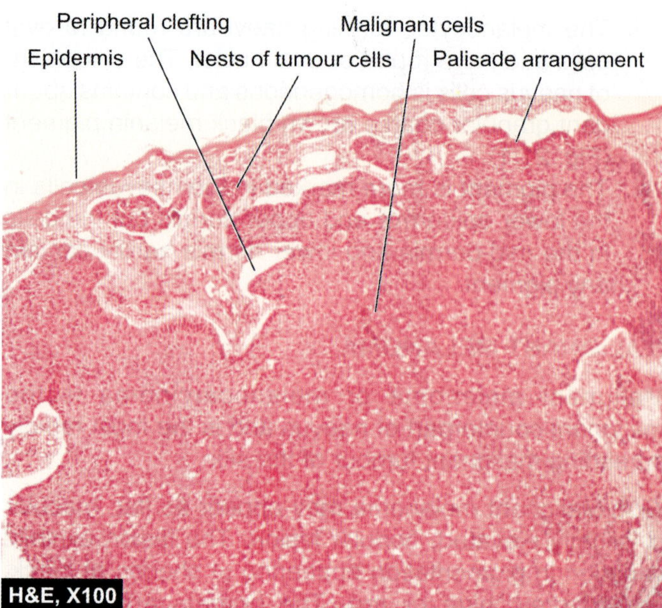

FIGURE 21.4: Solid basal cell carcinoma. The dermis is invaded by irregular masses of basaloid cells with characteristic peripheral palisaded appearance.

BASAL CELL CARCINOMA

Basal cell carcinoma or rodent ulcer is a locally invasive slow-growing tumour of the skin of face in the middle-aged that rarely metastasises.

G/A The tumour is commonly a nodular growth with central ulceration (nodulo-ulcerative). The margins of the tumour are pearly white and rolled while the base shows ulceration and destruction of underlying tissues like a rodent.

M/E

i. The tumour cells resemble normal basal cell layer of the skin and grow downwards from the epidermis in a variety of patterns—solid masses, nests, islands, strands, keratotic masses, adenoid etc.
ii. All patterns of tumour cells have one common characteristic feature—the cells forming the periphery of tumour have parallel alignment or show palisading (basaloid cells).
iii. The tumour cells are basophilic with hyperchromatic nuclei (Fig. 21.4).
iv. Stroma shrinks away from epithelial tumour nests, creating clefts or shrinkage artefacts which help in differentiating it from the adnexal tumours.

Exercise

22

Non-epithelial and Metastatic Tumours

Objectives

- Learn common examples of primary benign and malignant non-epithelial tumours (e.g. fibroma, fibrosarcoma)* and metastatic deposits (metastatic carcinoma lymph node, metastatic sarcoma lung).
- Describe salient gross and microscopic features of these conditions.

FIBROMA

True fibromas are uncommon tumours in soft tissues. Many fibromas are actually examples of hyperplastic fibrous tissue rather than true neoplasms. Fibrous growths of the oral soft tissues are, however, very common. These are not true tumours (unlike intraoral fibroma and papilloma), but are instead inflammatory or irritative in origin.

G/A These are of variable size and are generally circumscribed. Cut section shows grey white parenchyma.

M/E Fibroma is a benign, often pedunculated and well-circumscribed tumour occurring on the body surfaces and mucous membranes. It is composed of fully matured and richly collagenous fibrous connective tissue (Fig. 22.1).

Following variants of fibromas are distinguished:

i. *Fibroma molle or fibrolipoma*, also termed soft fibroma, is similar type of benign growth composed of mixture of mature fibrous connective tissue and adult-type fat.
ii. *Elastofibroma* is a rare benign fibrous tumour located in the subscapular region. It is characterised by association of collagen bundles and branching elastic fibres.
iii. *Fibroepithelial polyps* occur due to irritation or chronic trauma. These are composed of reparative fibrous tissue, covered by a thin layer of stratified squamous epithelium.
iv. *Fibrous epulis* is a lesion occurring on the gingiva and is localised hyperplasia of the connective tissue following trauma or inflammation in the area. *Giant cell epulis* is a variant seen more commonly in females as reactive change to trauma; the lesion shows numerous osteoclast-like giant cells and vascular stroma.

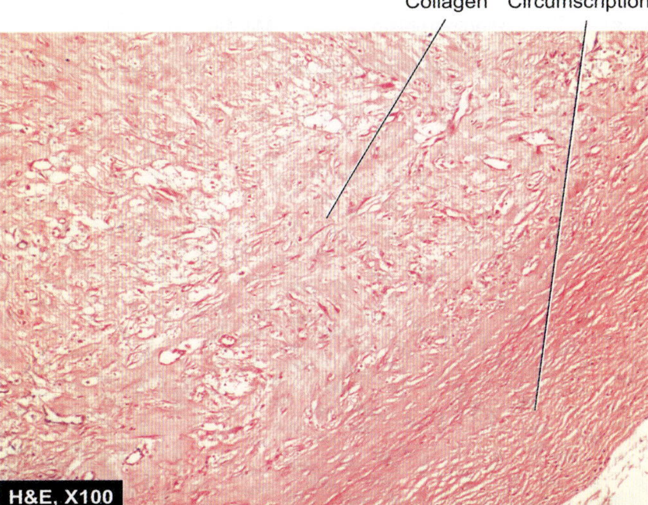

FIGURE 22.1: Fibroma of the oral cavity. The circumscribed lesion is composed of mature collagenised fibrous connective tissue.

*Examples of bone tumours are discussed in Exercise 25.

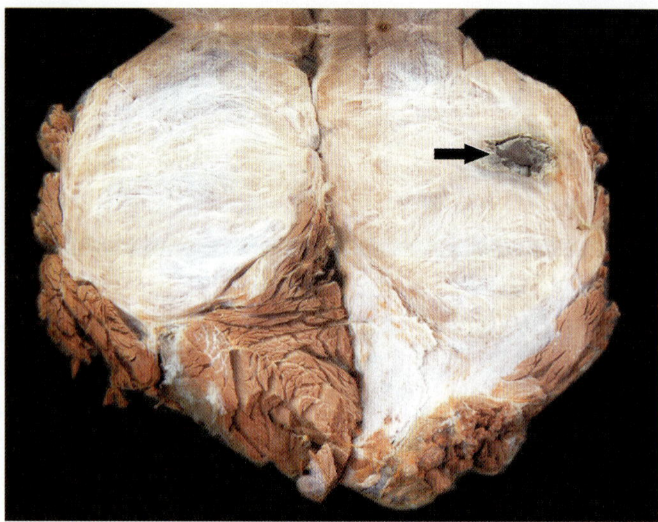

FIGURE 22.2: Soft tissue sarcoma. Sectioned surface shows an irregular and unencapsulated tumour invading muscle and has multiple nodularity and lobulations. Cut surface is grey-white fleshy with areas of haemorrhage (arrow) and necrosis.

FIBROSARCOMA

Fibrosarcoma is a slow-growing malignant tumour, affecting adults between 4th and 7th decades of life. Most common locations are the lower extremity (especially thigh and around the knee), upper extremity, trunk, head and neck, and retroperitoneum. The tumour is capable of metastasis, chiefly via the blood stream.

G/A Fibrosarcoma is a grey-white, firm, lobulated and characteristically circumscribed mass. Cut surface of the tumour is soft, fishflesh-like, with foci of necrosis and haemorrhages (Fig. 22.2).

M/E

i. The tumour is composed of uniform, spindle-shaped fibroblasts.
ii. These cells are arranged in intersecting fascicles. In well-differentiated tumours, such areas produce *'herring-bone pattern'* (herring-bone is a sea fish) (Fig. 22.3).
iii. Poorly-differentiated fibrosarcoma, however, has highly pleomorphic appearance with frequent mitoses and bizarre cells.

METASTATIC CARCINOMA LYMPH NODE

The regional lymph nodes may show metastatic deposits, most commonly from carcinomas but sometimes sarcomas may also metastasise to the regional lymph nodes.

G/A The affected lymph nodes are enlarged and matted. Cut surface shows homogeneous, grey-white deposits with areas of necrosis (Fig. 22.4).

M/E The features of metastatic carcinoma reproduce the picture of primary tumour. In a metastatic carcinoma from infiltrating duct carcinoma breast, the features are as under:

i. The nodal architecture is replaced by masses of malignant cells forming solid nests, cords and poorly-formed glandular structures.
ii. Part of cortex and capsule of the lymph node are intact (Fig. 22.5).

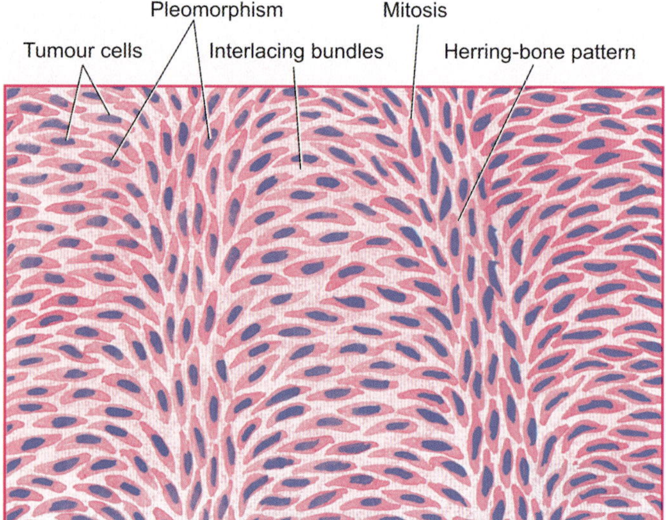

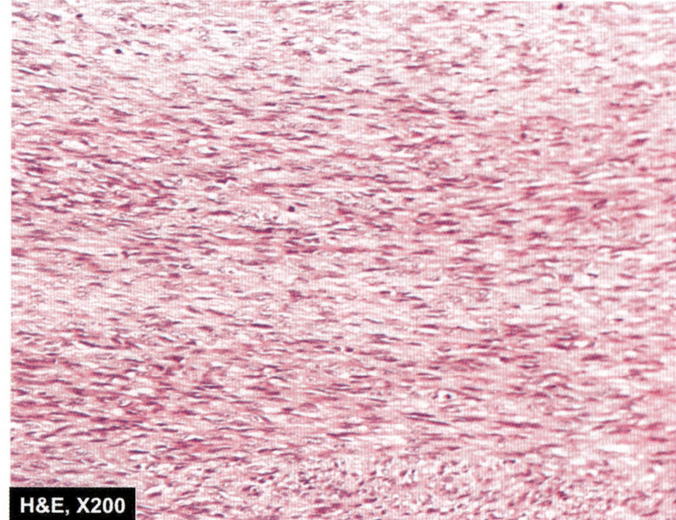

Figure 22.3: Fibrosarcoma. Microscopy shows a well-differentiated tumour composed of spindle-shaped cells forming interlacing fascicles producing a typical Herring-bone pattern. A few mitotic figures are also seen.

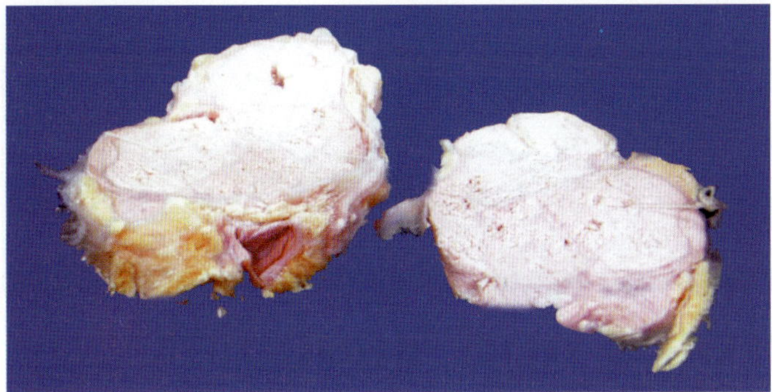

FIGURE 22.4: Metastatic carcinoma in lymph nodes. Matted mass of lymph nodes is surrounded by fat. Cut surface shows large irregular areas of grey-white colour replacing grey-brown nodal tissue.

METASTATIC SARCOMA LUNG

Sarcomas commonly metastasise through haematogeneous route to lungs, liver, bones, kidneys etc. Some carcinomas, however, too spread by haematogenous route.

G/A The metastatic nodules are scattered throughout all lobes of affected lung. The tumour nodules are circumscribed, soft and fleshy (Fig. 22.6).

M/E The metastatic tumour reproduces the picture of primary sarcoma. In metastatic deposits from malignant fibrous histiocytoma, the features are as under:

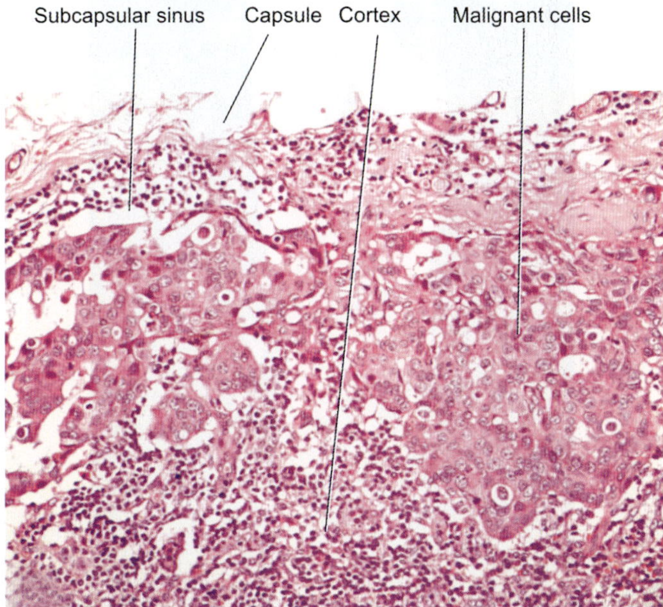

FIGURE 22.5: Metastatic carcinoma in lymph node. Lymphatic spread beginning by lodgement of tumour cells in subcapsular sinus via afferent lymphatics entering at the convex surface of the lymph node.

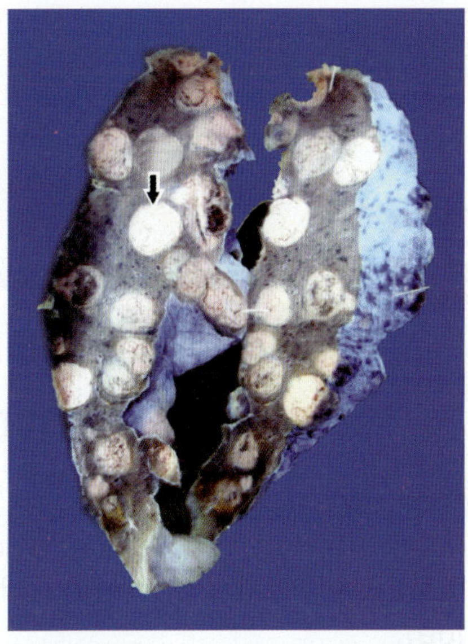

FIGURE 22.6: Metastatic sarcoma lung. Cut surface of the lung shows replacement of spongy parenchyma by multiple, variable-sized, circumscribed nodular masses (arrow). These masses are grey-white in colour and some show areas of haemorrhage and necrosis.

i. The tumour cells are pleomorphic and are oval to spindle-shaped.
ii. Multinucleate tumour giant cells are seen.
iii. The background may show myxoid material and areas of necrosis.
iv. There is generally rich vascularity (Fig. 22.7).

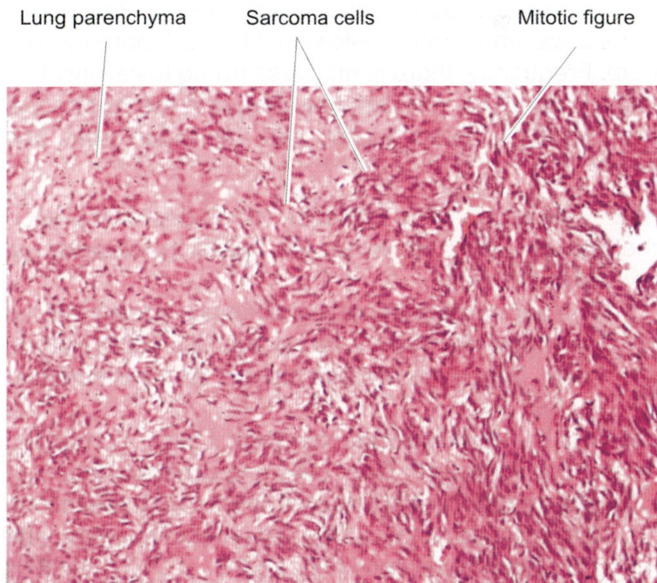

FIGURE 22.7: Metastatic sarcoma lung. Large mass of highly pleomorphic mesenchymal cells has replaced lung tissue on right.

Exercise

23 Atherosclerosis and Vascular Tumours

Objectives

- ⇨ Learn atheroma of the aorta and common examples of tumours of blood vessels (e.g. capillary haemangioma skin, cavernous haemangioma liver) and lymphatics (e.g. lymphangioma tongue).
- ⇨ Describe salient gross and microscopic features of these conditions.

ATHEROMA AORTA

A fully-developed atherosclerotic lesion is called atheromatous plaque or atheroma. It is located most commonly in the aorta (Fig. 23.1) and major branches of the aorta including coronaries.

G/A The plaque lesion is white to yellowish-white and may have ulcerated surface. Cut section shows firm *fibrous cap* and central yellowish-white soft porridge-like *core.* Frequently, there is grittiness owing to calcification in the lesion. The atheromatous plaque in the coronary is eccentrically located bulging into the lumen from one side.

M/E The appearance of plaque varies depending upon the age of lesion. However, the following features are invariably present:

i. The superficial luminal part of *fibrous cap* is covered by endothelium and is composed of smooth muscle cells, dense connective tissue and extracellular matrix.
ii. The cellular area under the fibrous cap is composed of macrophages, foam cells and lymphocytes.
iii. The deeper central soft *core* consists of extracellular lipid material, cholesterol clefts, necrotic debris and lipid-laden foam cells (Fig. 23.2).
iv. Calcium salts are deposited in the vicinity of necrotic area and in the lipid pool deep in the thickened intima (Fig. 23.3).

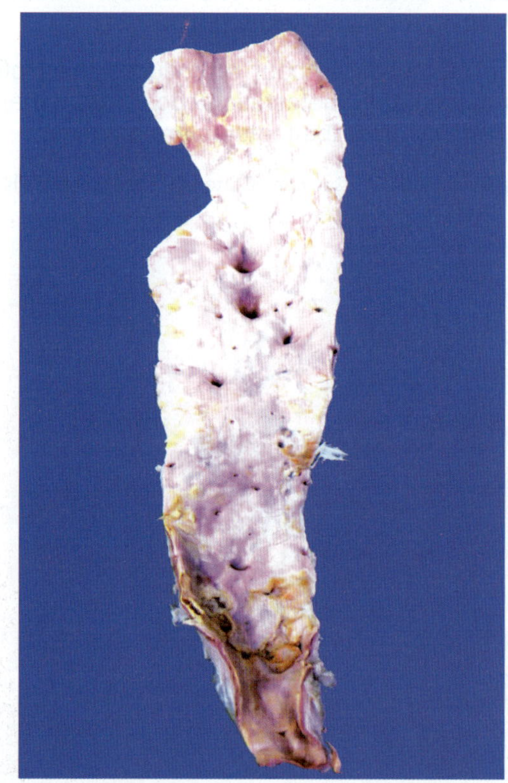

FIGURE 23.1: Fully-developed atheroma. The opened up aorta shows arterial branches coming out. The intimal surface shows yellowish-white lesions, slightly raised above the surface (arrow). A few have ulcerated surface. Many of these lesions are located near the ostial openings on the intima, thus partly occluding them.

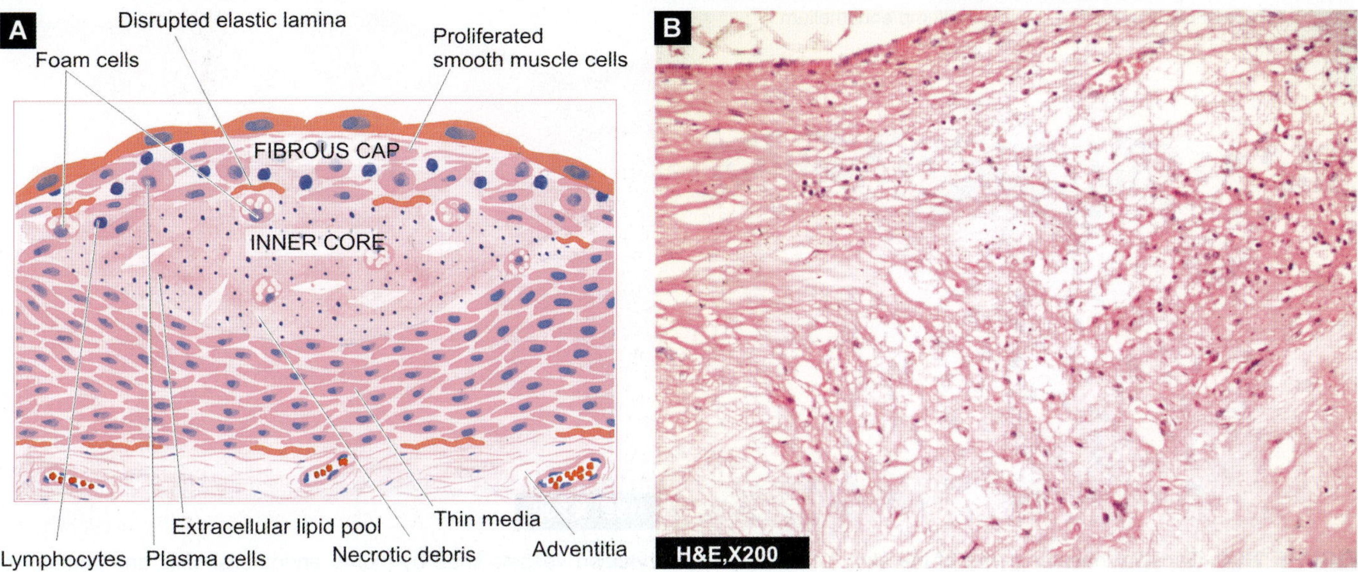

FIGURE 23.2: A, Diagrammatic view of the histologic appearance of a fully-developed atheroma. B, Atheromatous plaque showing fibrous cap and central core.

CAPILLARY HAEMANGIOMA SKIN

Haemangiomas are common lesions on the skin in infancy and childhood.

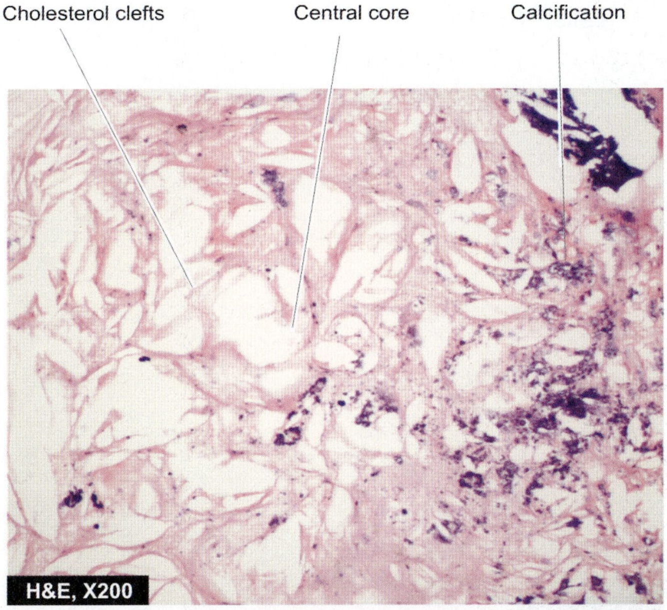

Cholesterol clefts
Central core
Calcification
H&E, X200

FIGURE 23.3: Complicated plaque lesion. There is critical narrowing of the coronary due to atheromatous plaque having dystrophic calcification.

G/A Haemangioma is a small or large, flat or slightly elevated, red to purple, soft and lobulated lesion varying in size from a few millimeters to a few centimeters in diameter.

M/E The lesion is well-defined but in the form of unencapsulated lobules.

i. The lobules are composed of capillary-sized, thin-walled, blood-filled vessels.
ii. The vessels are lined by single layer of plump endothelial cells surrounded by a layer of pericytes.
iii. Some stromal connective tissue separates lobules of blood vessels (Fig. 23.4).

CAVERNOUS HAEMANGIOMA LIVER

Cavernous haemangioma is a single or multiple, discrete or diffuse, soft and spongy mass.

G/A Cavernous haemangioma varies from 1 to 2 cm in diameter and is located in the organ in the form of red to blue, soft and spongy mass.

M/E

i. The lesion is composed of thin-walled cavernous vascular spaces, filled partly or completely with blood.
ii. The vascular spaces are lined by flattened endothelial cells.

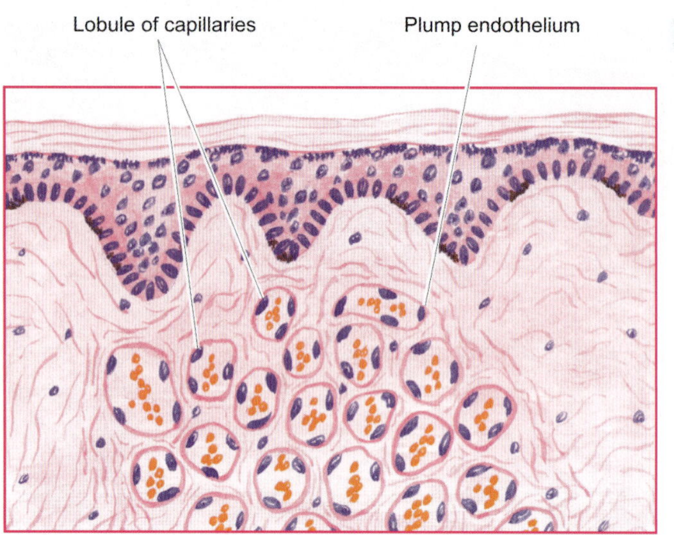

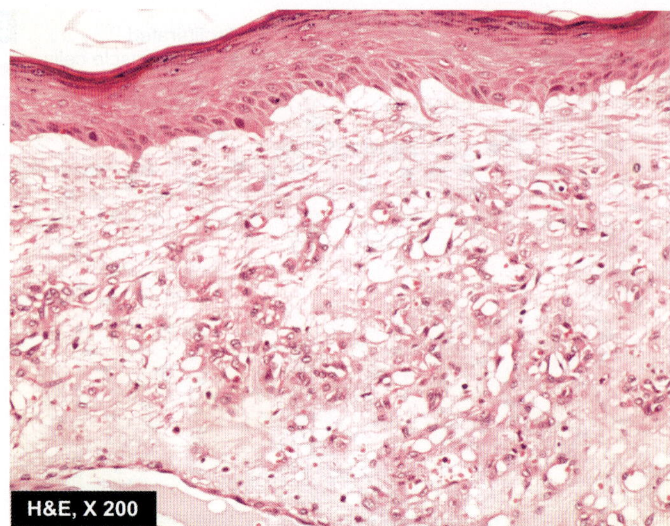

FIGURE 23.4: Capillary haemangioma of the skin. Lobules of capillary-sized vessels lined by plump endothelial cells and containing blood are lying in the dermis.

iii. The intervening stroma consists of scanty connective tissue (Fig. 23.5).

LYMPHANGIOMA TONGUE

Lymphangiomas are lymphatic counterparts of haemangioma and may be capillary or cavernous type, the latter being more common.

G/A Lymphangioma is a spongy mass which infiltrates the adjacent soft tissue diffusely.

M/E

i. There are large dilated lymphatic spaces containing homogeneous pink lymph fluid.
ii. These spaces are lined by flattened endothelial cells.

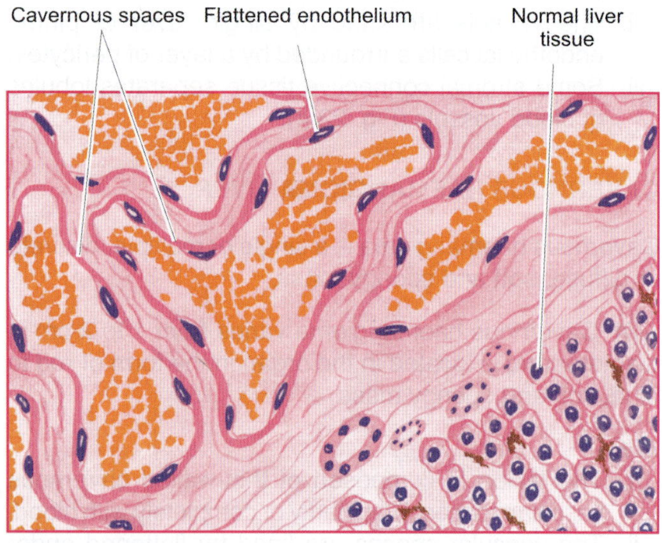

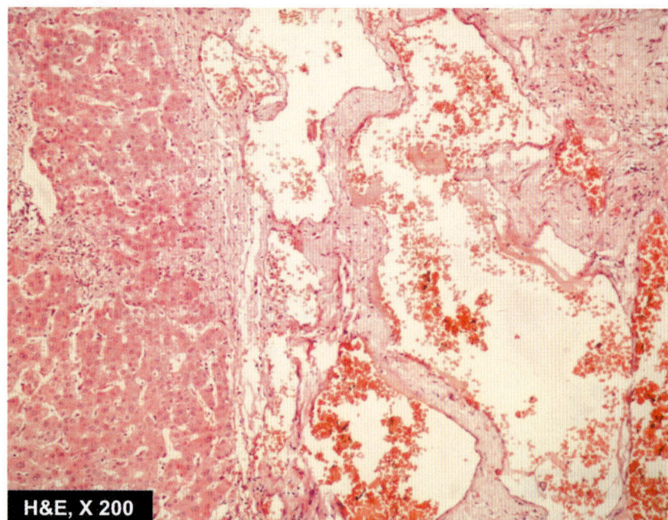

FIGURE 23.5: Cavernous haemangioma of the liver. Large cavernous spaces containing blood are seen in the liver tissue. Scanty connective tissue stroma is seen between the cavernous spaces.

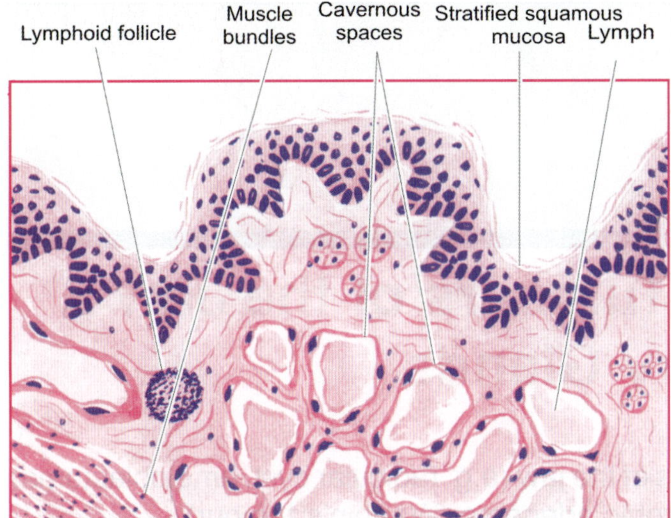

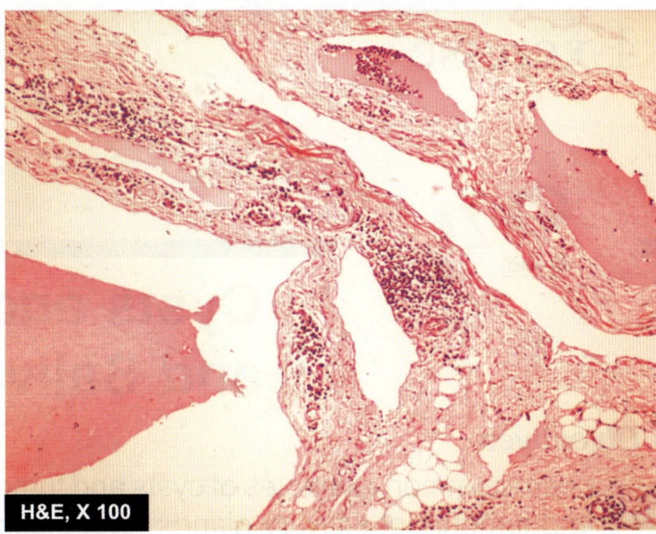

FIGURE 23.6: Cavernous lymphangioma of the tongue. Large cystic spaces lined by the flattened endothelial cells and containing lymph are present. Stroma shows scattered collection of lymphocytes.

iii. The intervening stromal tissue consists of connective tissue and lymphoid infiltrate, sometimes lymphoid follicles.

iv. Skeletal muscle bundles are present in the intervening stroma showing infiltration of the lesion into the muscle (Fig. 23.6).

Exercise

24

Cysts and Tumours of the Jaw and Salivary Glands

Objectives

- Learn common examples of cysts and tumours of the jaw (e.g. radicular cyst, ameloblastoma) and tumours of salivary glands (e.g. pleomorphic adenoma, Warthin's tumour).
- Describe salient gross and microscopic features of these conditions.

RADICULAR CYST

Radicular cyst, also called as apical, periodontal or dental cyst, is the most common cyst originating from the dental tissues. It arises consequent to inflammation following destruction of dental pulp such as in dental caries, pulpitis, and apical granuloma.

G/A Most often, radicular cyst is observed at the apex of an erupted tooth and sometimes contains thick pultaceous material.

M/E

i. The radicular cyst is lined by nonkeratinised squamous epithelium. Epithelial rete processes may penetrate the underlying connective tissues. Radicular cyst of the maxilla may be lined by respiratory epithelium.
ii. The cyst wall is fibrous and contains chronic inflammatory cells (lymphocytes, plasma cells with Russell bodies and macrophages) hyaline bodies and deposits of cholesterol crystals which may be associated with foreign body giant cells (Fig. 24.1).

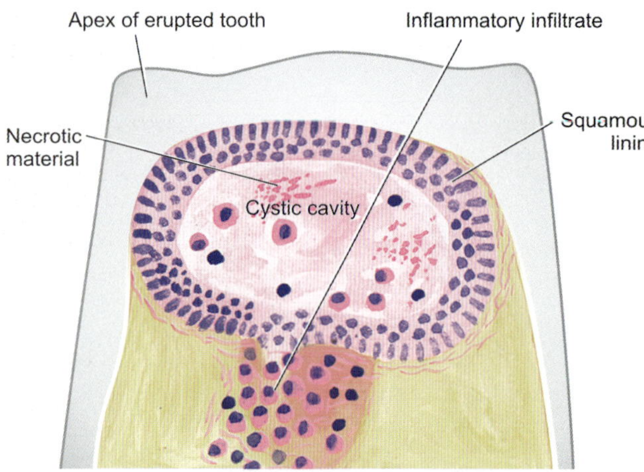

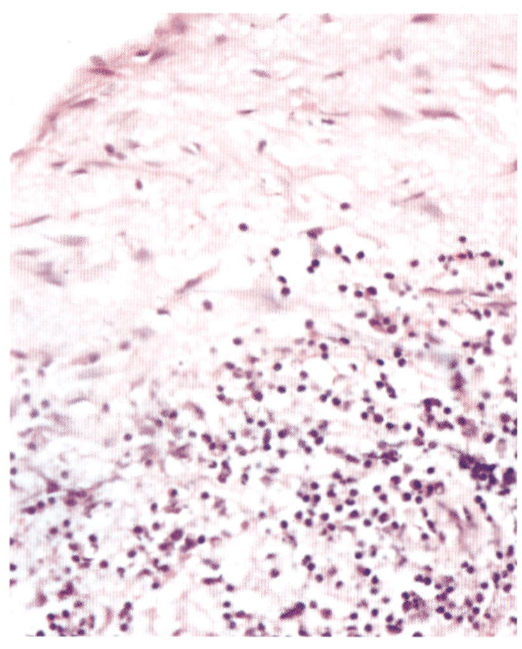

FIGURE 24.1: Dental (Radicular) cyst. The cyst wall is composed of fibrous tissue and is lined by non-keratinised squamous epithelium. The cyst wall is densely infiltrated by chronic inflammatory cells, chiefly lymphocytes, plasma cells and macrophages.

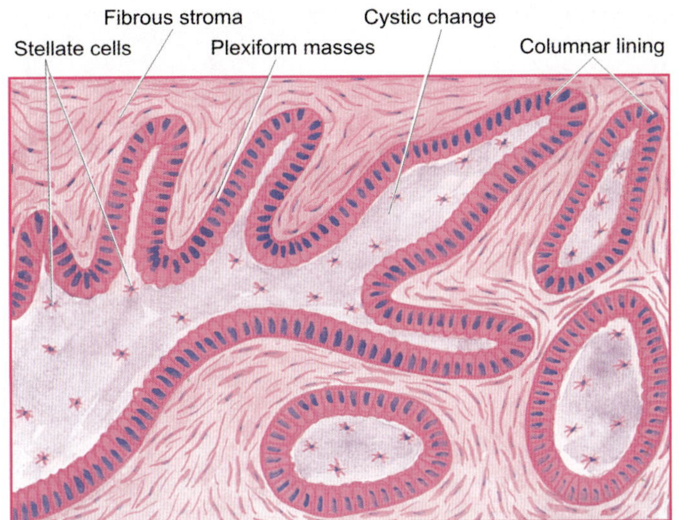

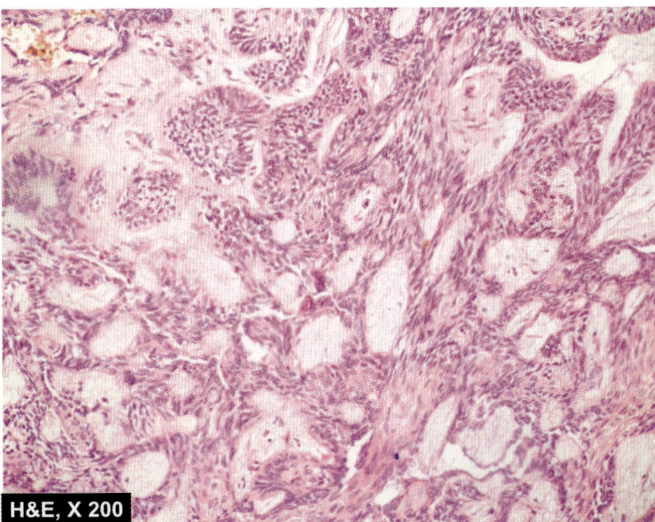

FIGURE 24.2: Ameloblastoma, follicular pattern. Epithelial follicles are seen in fibrous stroma. The follicles are composed of central area of stellate cells and peripheral layer of cuboidal or columnar cells. A few follicles show central cystic change .

AMELOBLASTOMA

Ameloblastoma is the common benign but locally aggressive epithelial odontogenic tumour, commonly in the mandible and maxilla.

G/A The tumour is grey-white, usually solid, sometimes cystic, replacing the affected bone.

M/E

i. Follicular pattern is the most common, characterised by follicles of varying size and shape which are separated by fibrous tissue.
ii. The follicles consist of central area of stellate cells and peripheral layer of cuboidal or columnar cells (Fig. 24.2).
iii. Other less common patterns include plexiform masses, acanthomatous pattern, basal cell pattern, and granular cell pattern.

PLEOMORPHIC ADENOMA

This is the commonest tumour in the parotid gland.

G/A The tumour is circumscribed, pseudoencapsulated, rounded and multilobulated, firm mass, 2-5 cm in diameter (Fig. 24.3). The cut surface is grey-white and bluish, variegated, with soft to mucoid consistency.

M/E The pleomorphic adenoma has two components: epithelial and mesenchymal (Fig. 24.4):

i. *Epithelial component* consists of various patterns like ducts, acini, tubules, sheets and strands of

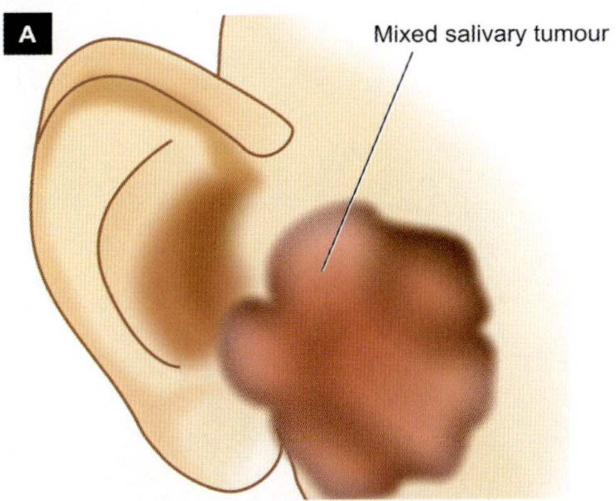

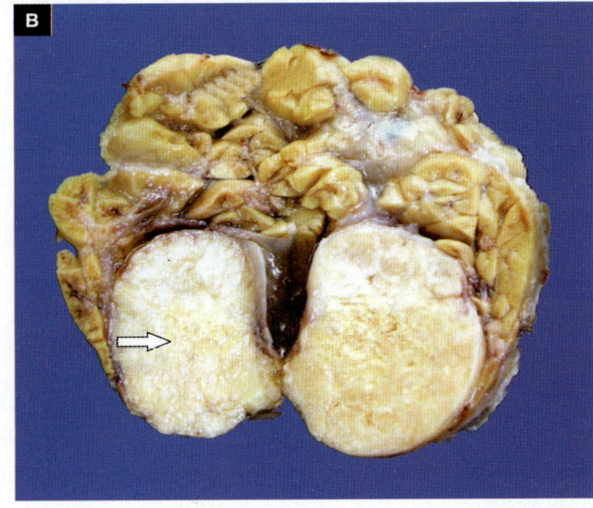

FIGURE 24.3: Pleomorphic adenoma (mixed salivary tumour) of the parotid gland. The salivary tissue is identified on section by lobules of soft tissue separated by thin septa. The cut surface of the tumour shows grey-white and light-bluish variegated semitranslucent parenchyma (arrow).

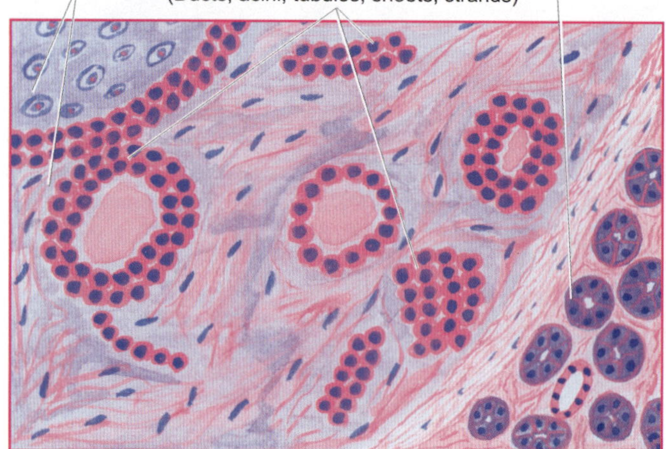

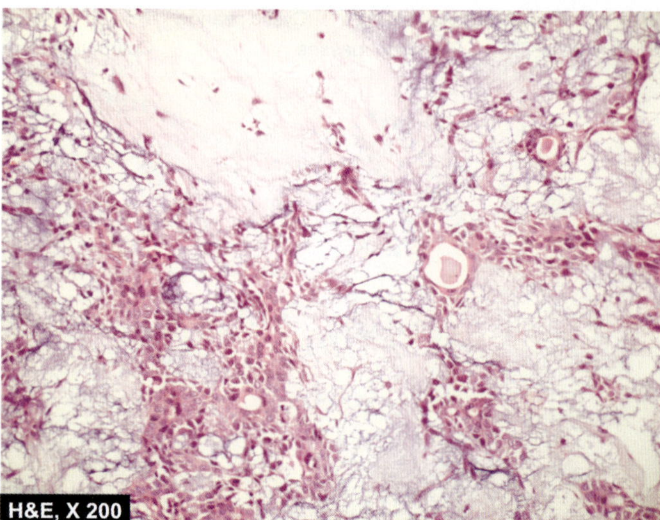

FIGURE 24.4: Pleomorphic adenoma, typical microscopic appearance. The epithelial element is composed of ducts, acini, tubules, sheets and strands of cuboidal and myoepithelial cells. These are seen randomly admixed with mesenchymal elements composed of pseudocartilage.

monomorphic cells of ductal or myoepithelial origin. These ductal cells are cuboidal or columnar while myoepithelial cells are polygonal or spindle-shaped.

ii. *Mesenchymal component* present in loose connective tissue includes myxoid, mucoid and chondroid matrix which simulates cartilage (pseudocartilage).

WARTHIN'S TUMOUR

Also given more descriptive names of papillary cystadenoma lymphomatosum and adenolymphoma, Warthin's tumour is a benign tumour of parotid gland arising from parotid ductal epithelium present in lymph nodes adjacent to or within parotid gland.

G/A The tumour is encapsulated and round to oval. Cut surface shows cystic spaces containing milky fluid and having papillary projections.

M/E The tumour shows 2 components (Fig. 24.5):

i. *Epithelial parenchyma* is composed of glandular and cystic structures having papillary arrangement and is lined by cells with eosinophilic cytoplasm.

ii. *Lymphoid stroma* is present as lymphoid tissue with germinal centres and is located under the epithelium.

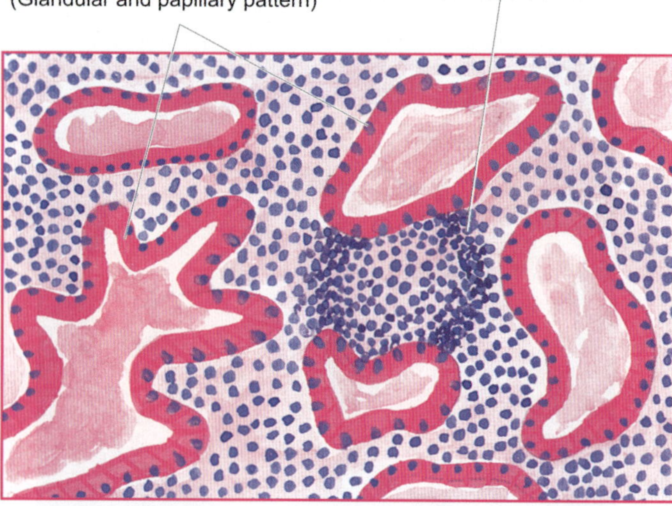

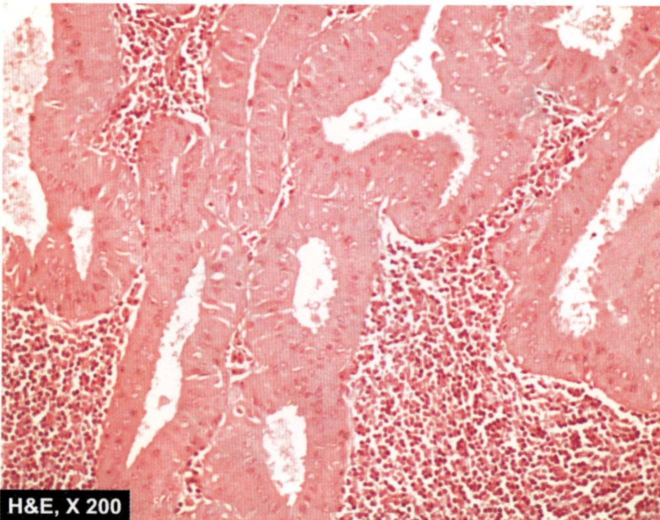

FIGURE 24.5: Warthin's tumour, showing eosinophilic epithelium forming glandular and papillary, cystic pattern with intervening stroma of lymphoid tissue.

Exercise

25 Common Diseases of Bones

Objectives

- ⇨ Learn common examples of inflammatory (e.g. chronic osteomyelitis, tuberculous osteomyelitis) and neoplastic (e.g. osteoclastoma, osteosarcoma) lesions of bones.
- ⇨ Describe salient gross and microscopic features of these conditions.

CHRONIC OSTEOMYELITIS

Chronic osteomyelitis is pyogenic or suppurative infection of the bone. Infection may occur by haematogenous route or by direct penetration or extension of bacteria.

G/A Residual and fragmented necrotic bone is seen as sequestrum while the surrounding reactive new bone is involucrum.

M/E

- i. There is marked mixed infiltrate of polymorphs and chronic inflammatory cells (lymphocytes, plasma cells and macrophages).
- ii. Chips of necrotic bone are seen in the pus.
- iii. Repair reaction consisting of osteoclasts, fibroblastic proliferation and new bone formation (Fig. 25.1).

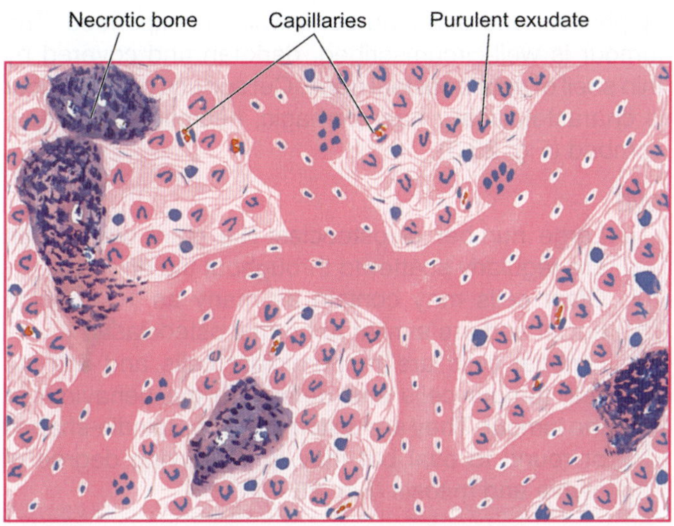

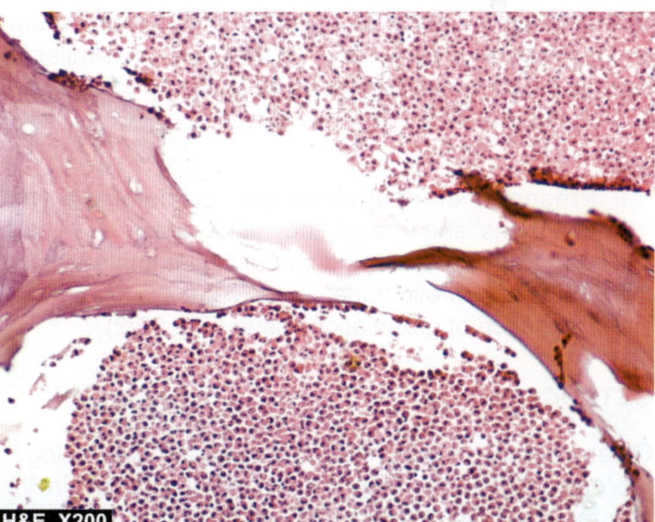

FIGURE 25.1: Chronic suppurative osteomyelitis. Histologic appearance shows necrotic bone and mixed inflammatory cells infiltrate of extensive purulent inflammatory exudates and inflammatory granulation tissue.

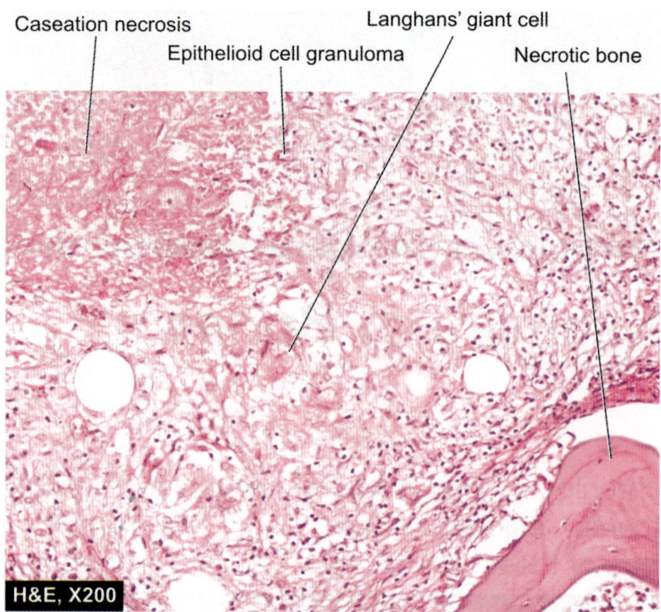

FIGURE 25.2: Tuberculous osteomyelitis consisting of epithelioid cell granulomas with minute areas of caseation necrosis and necrotic bone.

TUBERCULOUS OSTEOMYELITIS

Infection of the bone marrow by tubercle bacilli is a common condition in the underdeveloped and developing countries of the world. It occurs secondary to pulmonary tuberculosis by haematogenous spread. Tuberculosis of the vertebral bodies or Pott's disease is one of the important forms of tuberculous osteomyelitis.

G/A The appearance of necrotic bone (sequestrum) and surrounding new bone (involucrum) is similar to chronic osteomyelitis but foci of caseation necrosis may at times be evident.

M/E

i. Presence of epithelioid cell granulomas with Langhans' and foreign body giant cells.
ii. Admixture of acute and chronic inflammatory cells.
iii. Chips of necrotic bone.
iv. Formation of granulation tissue (Fig. 25.2).

OSTEOCLASTOMA

Osteoclastoma or giant cell tumour is a tumour arising in the epiphysis of the long bones, more common in the age range of 20 to 40 years. Common sites of involvement are: lower end of femur and upper end of tibia (i.e. about the knee), lower end of radius, and upper end of fibula.

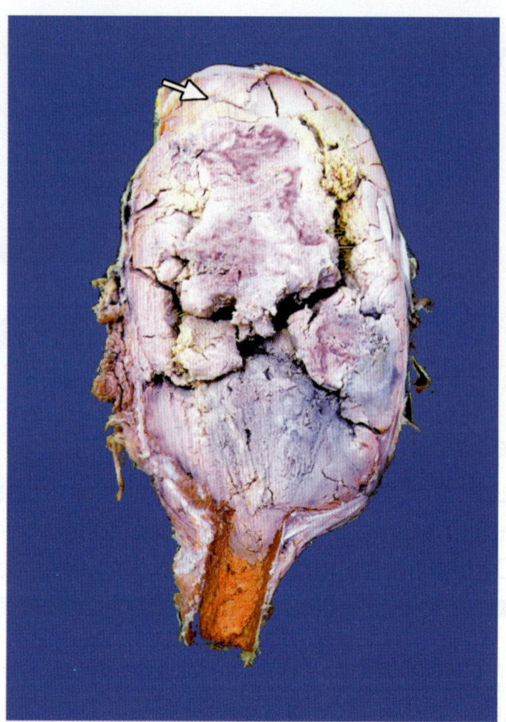

FIGURE 25.3: Giant cell tumour (osteoclastoma). The end of the long bone is expanded in the region of epiphysis (white arrow). Sectioned surface shows circumscribed, dark tan and necrotic tumour.

G/A Giant cell tumour is eccentrically located in the epiphyseal end of a long bone which is expanded. The tumour is well-circumscribed, dark-tan and covered by thin shell of subperiosteal bone. Cut surface of the tumour is characteristically haemorrhagic, necrotic and honeycombed (Fig. 25.3).

M/E

i. Large number of osteoclast-like giant cells which are regularly scattered throughout the stroma.
ii. Giant cells may contain as many as 100 benign nuclei and are similar to normal osteoclasts.
iii. Stromal cells are mononuclear cells and are the real tumour cells and determine the behaviour of the tumour. They are uniform, plump, spindle-shaped or round to oval but may have varying degree of atypia and mitosis (Fig. 25.4).

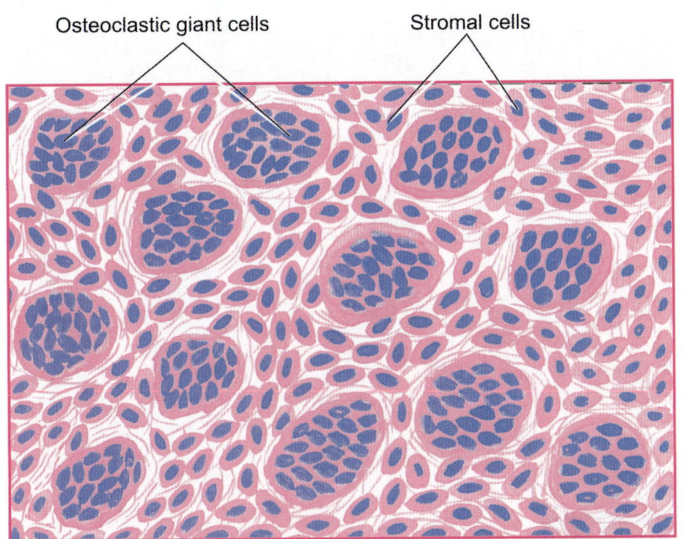

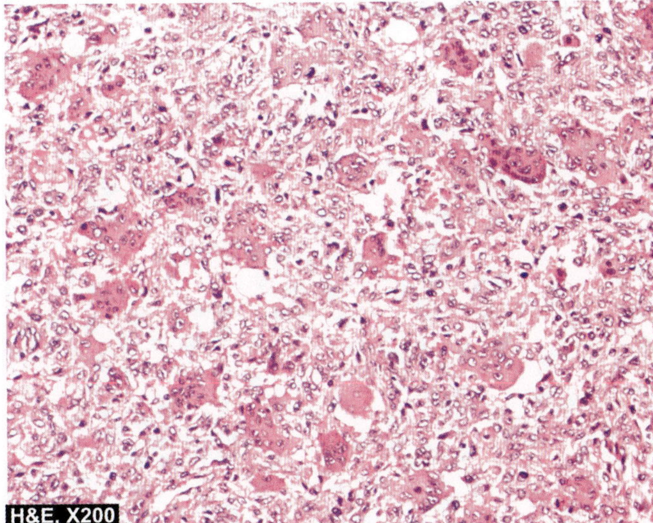

FIGURE 25.4: Osteoclastoma. The tumour shows spindle-shaped tumour cells, with uniformly distributed osteoclastic giant cells.

OSTEOSARCOMA

Osteogenic sarcoma or osteosarcoma is the most common primary malignant bone tumour. Classically, the tumour occurs in young patients between the age of 10 to 20 years. The tumour arises in the metaphysis of long bones, most commonly in the lower end of femur and upper end of tibia (i.e. around knee joint).

G/A The tumour appears as a grey-white, bulky mass at the metaphyseal end of a long bone of the extremity, generally sparing the articular end of the bone. Codman's triangle formed by the angle between lifting of periosteum and underlying surface of the cortex may be grossly identified. Cut surface of the tumour is grey-white with areas of haemorrhages and necrotic bone (Fig. 25.5).

M/E

i. *Sarcoma cells:* The tumour cells are anaplastic mesenchymal stromal cells which show marked pleomorphism and polymorphism i.e. variation in size as well as shape. The tumour cells may be spindled, round, oval, polygonal or bizarre tumour giant cells. They show hyperchromatism and atypical mitoses.
ii. *Osteogenesis:* The anaplastic sarcoma cells form osteoid matrix and bone directly, which lies interspersed in the areas of tumour cells (Fig. 25.6).

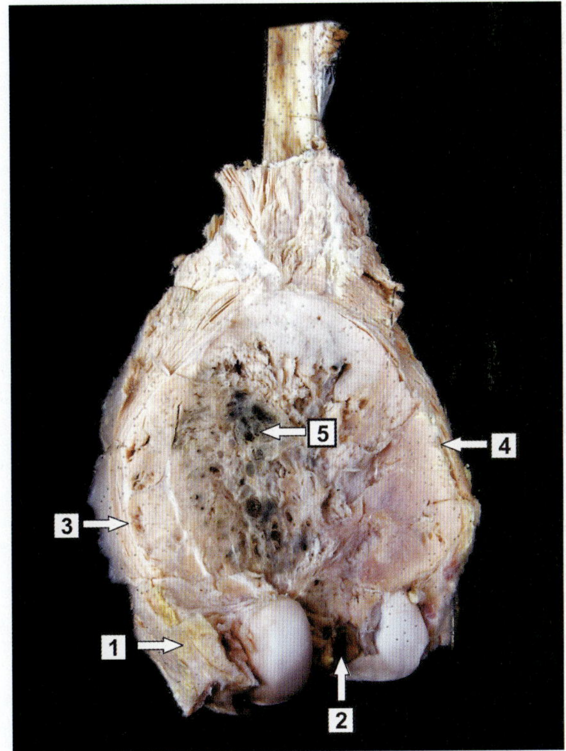

FIGURE 25.5: Osteosarcoma. The lower end of the femur shows a bulky expanded tumour in the region of metaphysis (1) sparing the epiphyseal cartilage (2). Sectioned surface of the tumour shows lifting of the periosteum by the tumour (3) and eroded cortical bone (4). Cut surface of the tumour is grey-white with areas of haemorrhage and necrosis (5).

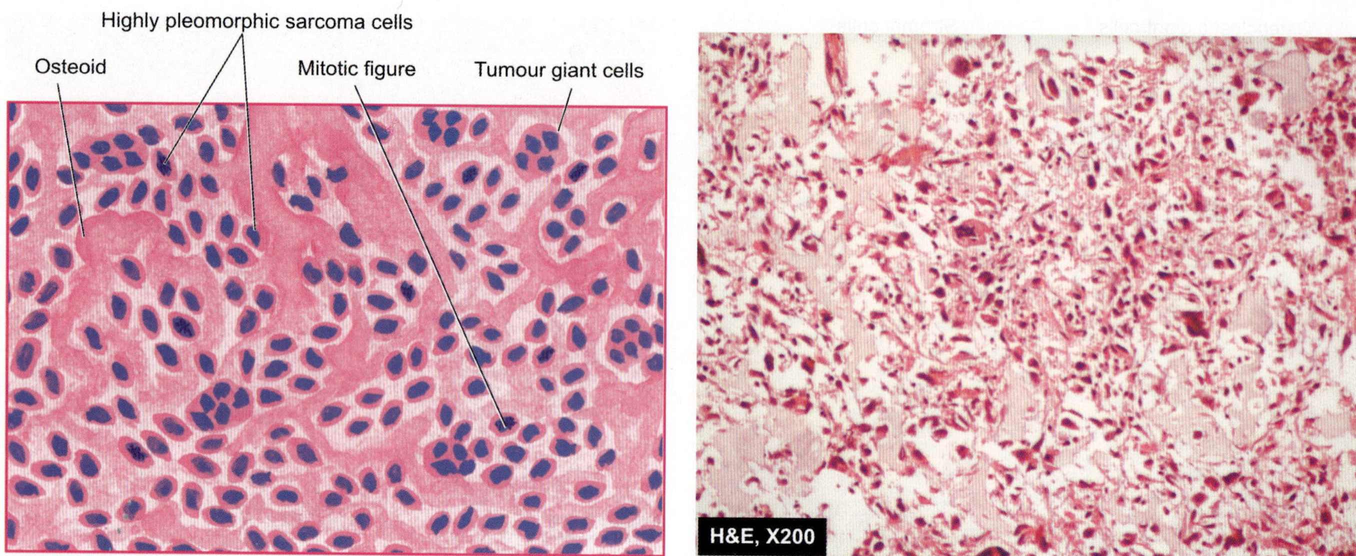

FIGURE 25.6: Osteosarcoma. The tumour cells show pleomorphic and polymorphic features with direct formation of osteoid by tumour cells.

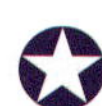

APPENDIX

Normal Values

Common and important normal values are given below under two main headings:

I. Weights and measurements of normal organs.
II. Laboratory values of clinical significance.

WEIGHTS AND MEASUREMENTS OF NORMAL ORGANS

In order to understand the significance of alterations in weight and measurement of an organ in disease, it is important to be familiar with the normal values. In the foregoing chapters, normal figures are given alongside the normal structure of each organ/system that precedes the discussion of pathologic states affecting it. Here, a comprehensive list of generally accepted normal weights and measurements of most of the normal organs in fully-developed, medium-sized individual are compiled in Table A-1.

Single value and value within brackets are indicative of the average figure for that organ. Measurements have been given as width × breadth (thickness) × length. An alphabetic order has been followed.

TABLE A-1: Weights and Measurements of Normal Organs.

Organ	*In Adults*
Brain:	
Weight (in males)	1400 gm
Weight (in females)	1250 gm
Volume of cerebrospinal fluid	120–150 ml
Heart:	
Weight (in males)	300–350 gm
Weight (in females)	250–300 gm
Thickness of right ventricular wall	0.3–0.5 cm
Thickness of left ventricular wall	1.3–1.5 cm
Circumference of mitral valve	10 cm
Circumference of aortic valve	7.5 cm
Circumference of pulmonary valve	8.5 cm
Circumference of tricuspid valve	12 cm
Volume of pericardial fluid	10–30 ml
Intestines:	
Length of duodenum	30 cm
Total length of small intestine	550–650 cm
Length of large intestine	150–170 cm
Kidneys:	
Weight each (in males)	150 gm
Weight each (in females)	135 gm
Liver:	
Weight (in males)	1400–1600 (1500) gm
Weight (in females)	1200–1400 (1300) gm
Lungs:	
Weight (right lung)	375–500 (450) gm
Weight (left lung)	325–450 (400) gm
Volume of pleural fluid	< 15 ml
Oesophagus:	
Length (cricoid cartilage to cardia)	25 cm
Distance from incisors to gastro-oesophageal junction	40 cm
Pancreas:	
Total weight	60–100 (80) gm

Contd...

TABLE A-1: Weights and Measurements of Normal Organs. (contd...)	
Organ	*In Adults*
Parotid glands:	
Weight (each)	30 gm
Pituitary gland (Hypophysis):	
Weight	500 mg
Placenta:	
Weight at term	400–600 gm
Prostate:	
Weight	20 gm
Spleen:	
Weight	125–175 (150) gm
Thymus:	
Weight	5–10 gm
Thyroid:	
Weight	15–40 gm

LABORATORY VALUES OF CLINICAL SIGNIFICANCE

Currently, the concept of 'normal values' and 'normal ranges' is replaced by 'reference values' and 'reference limits' in which the variables for establishing the values for the reference population in a particular test are well defined. Reference ranges are valuable guidelines for the clinician. However, the following cautions need to be exercised in their interpretation:

- *Firstly,* they should not be regarded as absolute indicators of health and ill-health since values for healthy individuals often overlap with values for persons afflicted with disease.
- *Secondly,* laboratory values may vary with the method and mode of standardisation used; reference ranges given below are based on the generally accepted values by the standard methods in laboratory medicine.
- *Thirdly,* although in most laboratories in the West and in all medical and scientific journals, international units (IU) conforming to the SI system are followed, but conventional units continue to be used in many laboratories in the developing countries of the world.

The WHO as well as International Committee for Standardisation in Haematology (ICSH) have recommended adoption of SI system by the scientific community throughout world. In this section, laboratory values are given in both conventional and international units. Conversion from one system to the other can be done as follows:

$$\text{mg/dl} = \frac{\text{mmol/L} \times \text{atomic weight}}{10}$$

$$\text{mmol/L} = \frac{\text{mg/dl} \times 10}{\text{atomic weight}}$$

According to the SI system, the prefixes and conversion factors for metric units of length, weight and volume are given in Table A-2.

TABLE A-2: Prefixes and Conversion Factors in SI System.

Prefix	*Prefix Symbol*	*Factor*	*Units of Length*	*Units of Weight*	*Units of Volume*
kilo-	k	10^3	kilometre (km)	kilogram (kg)	kilolitre (kl)
		1	metre (m)	gram (g)	litre (l)
deci-	d	10^{-1}	decimetre (dm)	decigram (dg)	decilitre (dl)
centi-	c	10^{-2}	centimetre (cm)	centigram (cg)	centilitre (cl)
milli-	m	10^{-3}	millimetre (mm)	milligram (mg)	millilitre (ml)
micro-	μ	10^{-6}	micrometre (μm)	microgram (μg)	microlitre (μl)
nano-	n	10^{-9}	nanometre (nm)	nanogram (ng)	nanolitre (nl)
pico-	p	10^{-12}	picometre (pm)	picogram (pg)	picolitre (pl)
femto-	f	10^{-15}	femtometre (fm)	femtogram (fg)	femtolitre (fl)
alto-	a	10^{-18}	altometre (am)	altogram (ag)	altolitre (al)

The laboratory values given here are divided into three sections: clinical chemistry of blood (Table A-3), other body fluids (Table A-4), and haematologic values (Table A-5). In general, an alphabetic order has been followed.

TABLE A-3: Clinical Chemistry of Blood.

Components	Fluid	Reference value	
		Conventional	*SI units*
Alcohol, ethyl	Serum/whole blood	Negative	Negative
mild to moderate intoxication		80-200 mg/dl	
marked intoxication		250-400 mg/dl	
severe intoxication		>400 mg/dl	
Aminotransferases (transaminases)			
aspartate (AST, SGOT)	Serum	12-38 U/L	0.20-0.65 µkat*/L
alanine (ALT, SGPT)	Serum	7-41 U/L	0.12-0.70 µkat/L
Bilirubin			
total	Serum	0.3-1.3 mg/dl	5.1-22 µmol/L
direct (conjugated)	Serum	0.1-0.4 mg/dl	1.7-6.8 µmol/L
indirect (unconjugated)	Serum	0.2-0.9 mg/dl	3.4-15.2 µmol/L
Blood volume			
total		60-80 ml/kg body weight	
red cell volume, males		30 ml/kg body weight	
females		25 ml/kg body weight	
Plasma volume, males		39 ml/kg body weight	
females		40 ml/kg body weight	
Calcium, total	Serum	8.7-10.2 mg/dl	2.2-2.6 mmol/L
Calcium, ionised	Whole blood	4.5-5.3 mg/dl	1.12-1.32 mmol/L
Chloride (Cl^-)	Serum	102-109 mEq/L	102-109 mmol/L
Cholesterol	Serum		
total desirable for adults		<200 mg/dl	<5.17 mmol/L
borderline high		200-239 mg/dl	5.17-6.18 mmol/L
high undesirable		≥240 mg/dl	>6.21 mmol/L
LDL-cholesterol, desirable range		<130 mg/dl	<3.34 mmol/L
borderline high		130-159 mg/dl	3.36-4.11 mmol/L
high undesirable		<160 mg/dl	>4.11 mmol/L
HDL-cholesterol, protective range		>60 mg/dl	>1.55 mmol/L
low		<40 mg/dl	<1.03 mmol/L
triglycerides		<160 mg/dl	<2.26 mmol/L
CO_2 content	Plasma	22-30 mEq/L (arterial)	22-30 mmol/L (arterial)
C-reactive proteins	Serum	0.2-3.0 mg/L	0.2-3.0 mg/L
Creatine kinase (CK), total	Serum		
males		51-294 U/L	0.87-5.0 µkat/L
females		39-238 IU/L	0.66-4.0 µkat/L
Creatine kinase-MB (CK-MB)	Serum	0-5.5 ng/ml	0-5.5 µg/L
Creatinine	Serum	0.6-1.2 mg/dl	53-106 µmol/L
Electrophoresis, protein	Serum	*See under proteins*	
Gamma-glutamyl transpeptidase (transferase) (γ-GT)	Serum	9-58 IU/L	0.15-1.00 µmol/L

*µkat (kat stands for katal, meaning catalytic activity) is a modern unit of enzymatic activity.

Contd...

TABLE A-3: Clinical Chemistry of Blood. *(contd...)*

Components	*Fluid*	*Reference value*	
		Conventional	*SI units*
Gases, arterial			
Bicarbonate (HCO_3^-)	Whole blood	22-30 mEq/L	22-30 mmol/L
pH	Whole blood	7.35-7.45	7.35-7.45
pCO_2	Whole blood	22-45 mmHg	4.3-6.0 kPa
pO_2	Whole blood	72-104 mmHg	9.6-13.8 kPa
Glucose (fasting)	Plasma		
normal		70-100 mg/dl	< 5.6 mmol/L
impaired fasting glucose (IFG)		101-125 mg/dl	5.6-6.9 mmol/L
diabetes mellitus		≥126 mg/dl	≥7.0 mmol/L
Glucose (2-hr post-prandial)	Plasma		
normal		<140 mg/dl	<7.8 mmol/L
impaired glucose tolerance (IGT)		140-200 mg/dl	7.8-11.1 mmol/L
diabetes mellitus		>200 mg/dl	>11.1 mmol/L
Haemoglobin A_{1C}	Whole blood	4-6%	0.04-0.06 Hb fraction
Immunoglobulins	Serum		
IgA		70-350 mg/dl	0.70-3.50 g/L
IgD		0-14 mg/dl	0-140 mg/L
IgE		<0.025 mg/dl	24-430 μg/L
IgG		700-1700 mg/dl	7.0-17.0 g/L
IgM		50-300 mg/dl	0.50-3.0 g/L
Lactate dehydrogenase (LDH)	Serum	115-221 U/L	2.0-3.8 μkat/L
Lactate/pyruvate ratio		10/1	
Lipase	Serum	3-43 U/L	0.51-0.73 μkat/L
Lipids	*See under cholesterol*		
Lipoproteins	Serum	0-30 mg/dl	0-300 mg/L
Oxygen (% saturation)			
arterial blood	Whole blood	94-100%	
venous blood	Whole blood	60-85%	
pH	Blood	7.35-7.45	7.35-7.45
Phosphatases			
acid phosphatase	Serum	0-5.5 U/L	0.90 μkat/L
alkaline phosphatase	Serum	33-96 U/L	0.56-1.63 μkat/L
Phosphorus, inorganic	Serum	2.5-4.3 mg/dl	0.81-1.4 mmol/L
Potassium	Serum	3.5-5.0 mEq/L	3.5-5.0 mmol/L
Prostate specific antigen (PSA)	Serum	0-4.0 ng/ml	0-4.0 μg/L
Proteins	Serum		
total		6.7-8.6 g/dl	67-86 g/L
albumin		3.5-5.5 g/dl (50-60%)	35-55 g/L
globulins		2.0-3.5 g/dl (40-50%)	20-35 g/L
A/G ratio		1.5-3 : 1	
Renal blood flow		1200 ml/min	
Rheumatoid factor	Serum	< 30 IU/ml	< 30 kIU/L
Sodium	Serum	136-146 mEq/L	136-146 mmol/L

Contd...

TABLE A-3: Clinical Chemistry of Blood. *(contd...)*			
		Reference value	
Components	*Fluid*	*Conventional*	*SI units*
Thyroid function tests			
radioactive iodine uptake (RAIU) 24-hr		5-30%	
thyroxine (T_4) total	Serum	5.4-11.7 µg/dl	70-151 nmol/L
triiodothyronine (T_3) total	Serum	77-135 ng/dl	1.2-2.1 nmol/L
thyroid stimulating hormone (TSH)	Serum	0.34-4.25 µIU/ml	0.34-4.25 mIU/L
Troponins, cardiac (cTn)			
troponin I (cTnI)	Serum	0-0.08 ng/ml	0-0.8 µg/L
troponin T (cTnT)	Serum	0-0.01 ng/ml	0-0.1 µg/L
Urea	Blood	20-40 mg/dl	3.3-6.6 mmol/L
Urea nitrogen (BUN)	Blood	7-20 mg/dl	2.5-7.1 mmol/L
Uric acid	Serum		
males		3.1-7.0 mg/dl	0.18-0.41 µmol/L
females		2.5-5.6 mg/dl	0.15-0.33 µmol/L

TABLE A-4: Other Body Fluids.			
		Reference value	
Components	*Fluid*	*Conventional*	*SI units*
Body volume, water			
total		50-70% (60%)	
intracellular		33%	
extracellular		27%	
interstitial fluid including lymph fluid		12%	
intravascular fluid or blood plasma		5%	
fluid in mesenchymal tissues		9%	
transcellular fluid		1%	
Cerebrospinal fluid (CSF)	CSF		
CSF volume		120-150 ml	
CSF pressure		60-150 mm water	
leucocytes		0-5 lymphocytes/ml	
pH		7.31-7.34	
glucose		40-70 mg/dl	
proteins		20-50 mg/dl	
FIGLU	24-hr urine	<3 mg/day	<17.2 µmol/day
Glomerular filtration rate (GFR)	Urine	180 L/day (about 125 ml/min)	
	4-15 mg/day		
Schilling's test (Intrinsic factor test)	24-hr urinary excretion	>10% of ingested dose of 'hot' vitamin B_{12}	
Urine examination	24-hr volume	600-1800 ml (variable)	
pH	Urine	5.0-9.0	
specific gravity, quantitative		Urine (random)	1.002-1.028 (average 1.018)
protein excretion	24-hr urine	<150 mg/day	

Contd...

TABLE A-4: Other Body Fluids. *(contd...)*

Components	*Fluid*	*Reference value*	
		Conventional	*SI units*
protein, qualitative	Urine (random)	Negative	
glucose excretion, quantitative	24-hr urine	50-300 mg/day	
glucose, qualitative	Urine (random)	Negative	
porphobilinogen	Urine (random)	Negative	
urobilinogen	24-hr urine	1.0-3.5 mg/day	
microalbuminuria (24-hour)		0-30 mg/24 hr	0-0.03 g/day
		(0-30 μg/mg creatinine)	(0-0.03 g/g creatinine)
Urobilinogen	Urine (random)	Present in 1: 20 dilution	

TABLE A-5: Normal Haematologic Values.

Components	*Fluid*	*Reference value*	
		Conventional	*SI units*
Erythrocytes and Haemoglobin			
Erythrocyte count	Blood		
males		4.5-6.5 × 10^{12}/L (mean 5.5 × 10^{12}/L)	
females		3.8-5.8 × 10^{12}/L (mean 4.8 × 10^{12}/L)	
Erythrocyte diameter		6.7-7.7 mm (mean 7.2 μm)	
Erythrocyte thickness			
peripheral		2.4 μm	
central		1.0 μm	
Erythrocyte indices (Absolute values)	Blood		
mean corpuscular haemoglobin (MCH)		27-32 pg	
mean corpuscular volume (MCV)		77-93 fl	
mean corpuscular haemoglobin concentration (MCHC)		30-35 g/dl	
Erythrocyte life-span	Blood	120±30 days	
Erythrocyte sedimentation rate (ESR)	Blood		
Westergren 1st hr, males		0-15 mm	
females		0-20 mm	
Wintrobe, 1st hr, males		0-9 mm	
females		0-20 mm	
Ferritin	Serum		
males		30-250 ng/ml	30-250 μg/L
females		10-150 ng/ml	10-150 μg/L
Folate			
body stores		2-3 mg	
daily requirement		100-200 μg	
red cell level	Red cells	150-450 ng/ml	340-1020 nmol/L
serum level	Serum	6-18 ng/ml	12-40 nmol/L
Free erythrocyte protoporphyrin (FEP)	Red cells	20 μg/dl	
Haematocrit (PCV)	Blood		
males		40-54%	0.47 ± 0.07 L/L
females		37-47%	0.42 ± 0.05 L/L

Contd...

TABLE A-5: Normal Haematologic Values. *(contd...)*			
		Reference value	
Components	*Fluid*	*Conventional*	*SI units*
Haemoglobin (Hb)			
adult haemoglobin (HbA)	Whole blood		
males		13.0-18.0 g/dl	130-180 g/L
females		11.5-16.5 g/dl	115-165 g/L
plasma Hb (quantitative)		0.5-5 mg/dl	5-50 mg/L
haemoglobin A_2 (HbA_2)		1.5-3.5%	
haemoglobin, foetal (HbF) in adults		<1%	
HbF, children under 6 months		<5%	
Iron, total	Serum	40-140 μg/dl	7-25 μmol/L
total iron binding capacity (TIBC)	Serum	250-406 μg/dl	45-73 μmol/L
iron saturation	Serum	20-45% (mean 33%)	0.20-0.45
Iron intake		10-15 mg/day	
Iron loss			
males		0.5-1.0 mg/day	
females		1-2 mg/day	
Iron, total body content			
males		50 mg/kg body weight	
females		35 mg/kg body weight	
Iron, storage form (ferritin and haemosiderin)		30% of body iron	
Osmotic fragility	Blood		
slight haemolysis		at 0.45 to 0.39 g/dl NaCl	
complete haemolysis		at 0.33 to 0.36 g/dl NaCl	
mean corpuscular fragility		0.4-0.45 g/dl NaCl	
Reticulocytes	Blood		
adults		0.5-2.5%	
infants		2-6%	
Transferrin	Serum	200-400 mg/dl	2-4 g/L
Vitamin B_{12}			
body stores		10-12 mg	
daily requirement		2-4 μg	
serum level	Serum	280-1000 pg/ml	280-1000 pmol/L
Leucocytes			
Differential leucocyte count (DLC)	Blood film or CBC counter		
P (polymorphs or neutrophils)		40-75% (2,000-7,500/μl)	
L (lymphocytes)		20-50% (1,500-4,000/μl)	
M (monocytes)		2-10% (200-800/μl)	
E (eosinophils)		1-6% (40-400/μl)	
B (basophils)		< l% (10-100/μl)	
Total leucocyte count (TLC)	Blood		
adults		4,000-11,000/μl	
infants (full term, at birth)		10,000-25,000/μl	
infants (1 year)		6,000-16,000/μl	

Contd...

TABLE A-5: Normal Haematologic Values. *(contd...)*			
		Reference value	
Components	*Fluid*	*Conventional*	*SI units*
Platelets and Coagulation			
Bleeding time (BT)			
Ivy's method	Prick blood	2-7 min	
template method		2.5-9.5 min	
Clot retraction time	Clotted blood		
qualitative		Visible in 60 min (complete in <24-hr)	
quantitative		48-64% (55%)	
Clotting time (CT)	Whole blood		
Lee and White method		4-9 min at 37°C	
Euglobin lysis time		72 hr	
Fibrinogen	Plasma	200-400 mg/dl	2-4 g/L
Fibrin split (or degradation) products (FSP or FDP)	Plasma	<10 μg/ml	<10 mg/L
Partial thromboplastin time with kaolin (PTTK) or activated partial thromboplastin time (APTT)	Plasma	30-40 sec	
Platelet count	Blood	150,000-400,000/μl	
Prothrombin time (PT) (Quick's one-stage method)	Plasma	10-14 sec	
Thrombin time (TT)	Plasma	<20 sec (control ± 2 sec)	

Index

*The letter "**t**" after page number in the index below denotes Table and the letter "**f**" stands for Figure on that page.*